Vertigo

Shabih H. Zaidi • Arun Sinha

Vertigo

A Clinical Guide

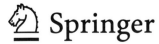 Springer

Shabih H. Zaidi
Department of ENT and Audiology
City Hospital
Birmingham
UK

Arun Sinha
Department of ENT and Audiology
City Hospital
Birmingham
UK

ISBN 978-3-642-36484-6   ISBN 978-3-642-36485-3   (eBook)
DOI 10.1007/978-3-642-36485-3
Springer Heidelberg New York Dordrecht London

Library of Congress Control Number: 2013942464

Printed on acid-free paper

Springer is part of Springer Science+Business Media (www.springer.com)

*Lovingly dedicated to our parents
and our families*

Foreword

The care provided to patients with disorders of balance has in recent years undergone a welcome and long overdue renaissance. Many factors have had a role in this enhanced delivery of healthcare to these individuals. There has been the recognition of new disorders and the re-evaluation of the investigation and treatment of those of which we are more familiar. Improved understanding of the interpretation of the results of investigations of the balance pathway has aided the diagnostic process. Our colleagues in radiology have more accurately defined conditions of the inner ear and central pathways to further aid in diagnosis. We now better understand the roles of rehabilitation and surgery, and improved quality of reporting of the outcomes of our interventions places us in a position whereby patient counseling is now a more accurate science.

Despite these innovations and the application of new technology perhaps the greatest contributor to improved outcomes has been the changes in the way we deliver our balance services and the development of the team approach. With an ageing population the demand for balance services will continue to grow exponentially, and it falls largely to clinicians to develop efficient and cost-effective approaches to provide this.

The balance patient is, in my view, best managed by multidisciplinary teams, working in dedicated balance clinics that have specialist knowledge and expertise. This expertise can only be obtained by a combination of high quality training in the clinical arena combined with a thorough understanding of the knowledge base. Within the pages of this book the attentive reader will find all that is required to equip themselves with this necessary knowledge and understanding. I hope this will inspire some to develop high quality services for their local populations and maybe also stimulate a thirst for further research in this highly rewarding and extremely important subject.

Richard M. Irving, MD, FRCS
Consultant Neuro-otologist, Skull Base Surgeon,
Queen Elizabeth, University Hospital,
Birmingham, UK

Preface

Medicine is a lifetime profession, and we the lifelong learners. Not a day goes by when we do not learn something new. We have spent several decades in Otolaryngology, learning, sharing and teaching. Otology has dominated our lives for many long years, and we have seen sea changes in this speciality. We continue to serve our patients with the latest knowledge and matching skills.

We have gained much through our long association with various universities and teaching hospitals in many parts of the world. The NHS, UK, is our nursery, to which we owe much and continue to benefit with its rich and invaluable resources. We see a large number of patients at the various hospitals of our trust, affiliated to the University of Birmingham and the West Midlands Deanery.

For many years, we have been engaged in research on the subject of vertigo. It is a fascinating and mind-boggling subject indeed. Numerous textbooks are available for an avid reader to benefit from. Besides, in today's age of communication, particularly due to the electronic media, one can never starve of the lack of information on any subject. Vertigo is no exception. We have attempted to look at its many facets from a clinician's view point. There is much to learn as there are huge gaps in our knowledge base. We fully comprehend our shortcomings. We simply wish to share our experience with our colleagues. We would also certify that observing the principle of confidentiality all clinical data is duly anonymised.

An audio-vestibular service is an absolute necessity for the investigation of vertigo. We are blessed with an excellent lab. Dr. Suki Dhillon and her team, particularly Phil, Phil Y.S, Parmajeet, Mark, Helen, Sameer, Rashcida, Jag and Carl, helped us immensely. We are grateful to them all.

We would particularly like to thank Claire Danks who helped us with the VNGs and vestibular investigations. Her contribution is immeasurable. Karen Harris deserves special thanks for helping us out with the interpretations of some VNGs. Kathy, Tammy and Tracy also deserve to be acknowledged.

No medical documentation is possible without an excellent library and referencing service. We want to acknowledge the support given us by the librarians of the City and Sandwell hospitals, particularly Sally, Nicola, Angela, Cheryl and Stacey. We must duly acknowledge the support of our nursing colleagues, Marion, Santosh, Martin, Connie, Ann, Diane, Sam, Lorraine, Michelle and Dawn. We also wish to thank the medical director and the executive authority of Sandwell and West Birmingham NHS trust for allowing the use of the services. And last but not least, a note of gratitude to our editor Sylvana Freyberg, and Springer, for publishing our humble work.

Birmingham, UK   Shabih H. Zaidi
                                                                                    Arun Sinha

Contents

Part I

Fundamentals

Nomenclature and Epidemiology

Vertigo is a malady for all ages. It is an enigma. It is also a common clinical condition seen by physicians of many specialties on almost daily basis. The word vertigo originates from a Latin word 'vertere' which means 'to turn'. It has no specific definition *per se*. Being a broad-based entity, it has been defined in more than one ways. Perhaps the commonest definition is that it is a 'subjective sense of movement of objects'. It has also been called a 'hallucination of movement' and even a 'false sense of movement of things and people'. Perhaps the most suitable definition could be 'an illusion of movement'. It basically implies that as long as the movement described by the patient is in his perception and not physically present, it may be called vertigo. It is a 'perception and not a reality'.

The hearing and equilibrium committee of the American Academy of ORL – Head and Neck Surgery gave a definition, which is generally accepted as a standard definition. They defined Vertigo as the 'sensation of motion when on motion is occurring relative to earth's gravity' (Committee on Hearing and Equilibrium 1995).

Vertigo may be rotational, oscillating or tilting in nature. Being a subjective sensation, all kinds of descriptions may be given by the patients. As long as a movement does not actually exist, it may be defined as vertigo. Like many other medical entities, the debate over the exact definition of vertigo may continue for quite some time to come. Suffice it to say though that from a clinician's point of view, a broad description of 'subjective sensation of movement of objects' is good enough to serve the purpose.

Vertigo is classified as either peripheral or central. The vestibular causes are included in the peripheral category and those related to central nervous system belong to the central category. Some of the common causes will be discussed later on.

But is dizziness the same as vertigo? Can the term 'balance disorders' or simply 'imbalance' be substituted for vertigo, giddiness or dizziness, etc.? Well academicians can look into these nuances of words and the semantics at length. By and large most clinicians and audio-vestibular scientists will be happy to get along with the diagnosis and the management once they are satisfied that what the patient has

S.H. Zaidi, A. Sinha, *Vertigo*,
DOI 10.1007/978-3-642-36485-3_1, © Springer-Verlag Berlin Heidelberg 2013

described is a true and genuine 'feeling of perception of movement of objects without the real existence of such a movement'.

Light-headedness is often confused with dizziness and vertigo. One should be quite clear about it. Light-headedness is actually a fleeting sensation of unsteadiness as if one is about to drop down. It is often experienced by the cardiac patients with poor cardiac compensation, who may sometimes develop a state of pre syncope. It is actually brought about by the decline in the cerebral perfusion and is usually noticed on a physical activity such as rising from a chair. Being a momentary sensation it disappears shortly leaving no squeal behind. Of course in a more severe variety, one may collapse, which is a different matter altogether demanding a thorough investigation and due management.

Dizziness is perhaps closest to the definition of vertigo, though some experts have called it disequilibrium as if one is standing on a moving boat. The intensity of dizziness may vary and can in fact lead to more intense feeling of the objective movement of elements around the subject; hence, the mimicry with vertigo.

Another condition seen in balance clinics is called oscillopsia. It is best described as the sense of stationary objects in motion. It is obviously an illusionary state and must not be confused with the classical vertigo caused by vestibular disease, though it can be induced by stimulation of the vestibular system. In such situations it is usually the result of the failure of the quintessential vestibulo-ocular reflex to lead to a suitable ocular movement in compensation for a head movement. The image thus falling onto retina with the movement of head leads to an ocular movement which can be seen.

This clinical guide is designed to cover the fundamentals of applied anatomy and physiology of balance. It will also cover the salient clinical conditions that contribute to the major bulk of disease causing significant impact on the patient's day-to-day life. Relevant diagnostic tests carried out in our laboratory will be described, followed by documentation of many interesting clinical cases that we have encountered in our practice in the last 5 years. The management of some cases will obviously be discussed at some length followed by a narration of the current and future trends in the diagnosis, care and management of these patients.

The epidemiology of vertigo is difficult to define and measure with absolute certainty, as it is a non-palpable, non-tangible, only a sensual feeling with limited signs to be employed as evidence.

The incidence and prevalence of vertigo vary from country to country and region to region. Many factors may influence the epidemiology of vertigo in a given population. For instance, in a younger population its incidence is lower than in an ageing population. Likewise, many nations have higher prevalence of underlying metabolic conditions like diabetes and hypertension that would impact the final picture of the epidemiology of vertigo. As we shall discuss later on, the major emphasis in this book rests upon vestibular causes of vertigo; however, one has to sift through a plethora of information and filter out the genuine vestibular pathologies from a whole range of other conditions that the patient may possess.

The literature search is the founding brick of any medical writing. In order to understand the nuances of a clinical condition, one must know its epidemiology, its pattern, presentation, impact and management. So we performed a comprehensive survey of most of these elements, and after excluding the relatively less important material, we chose some that are relevant and contemporary. They are included here.

In the field of epidemiology of vertigo, Neuhauser shines above all. His work is thorough, scientifically sound, technically flawless and highly informative. Some of his studies are mentioned here to let the reader have a flavour of the prevalence, incidence and characteristic presentation of various components that join together to compose this clinical entity called vertigo.

Neuhauser (2009) performed a population-based study, which is one of the most authentic sources of epidemiology, often quoted in the literature. It showed that the lifetime prevalence of vestibular vertigo was 7.4 %, the 1-year prevalence was 4.9 % and the incidence was 1.4 %. Numerous other similar studies duly informs us that the vestibular vertigo is common in the general population, affecting approximately 5 % of adults in 1 year. It is believed that the frequency and health-care impact of vestibular symptoms at the population level (Global Burden of Disease) have been underestimated. Many patients do not consult a physician and treat themselves with over-the-counter drugs. Suffice it to say it can be harmful and must not be encouraged. According to this survey, however, 80 % of vertigo patients consulted a physician due to the intensity of vertigo.

Besides, interruption of daily activities and co-morbidity in the form of tinnitus, depression and several cardiovascular diseases were also recorded. We agree with this study and strongly believe that vertigo is often the cause of misery not just because it is crippling but also due to co-morbidities that often accompany it, particularly in a certain age group. Vertigo was described as a rotational movement, a sense of movement of objects, provided such as movement actually does not exist.

Lempert and Neuhauser (2008) looked at the prevalence of some of these conditions. They agreed that migraine and vertigo are common in the general population with lifetime prevalence of about 16 % for migraine and 7 % for vertigo. Therefore, they believe that a concurrence of the two conditions can be expected in about 1.1 % of the general population by chance alone. However, they noted that recent epidemiological evidence suggested that the actual co-morbidity was higher (3.2 %). They attempted to explain on the basis that dizziness occurred more frequently in migraine sufferers than in controls. In addition, they also noted an increasing recognition of a syndrome called vestibular migraine (VM), which is 'vertigo directly caused by migraine'. They believed that it affected more than 1 % of the general population, about 10 % of patients in dizziness clinics and at least 9 % of patients in migraine clinics.

This particular paper by Neuhauser and Lempert gives so much information about various aspects of vertigo, right from the epidemiology to the impact on human health, that we are obliged to call this paper worthy of enormous credentials for its content and worthiness related to vertigo. It is highly recommended for our reader to consult. Many subjects that these two authors have discussed match with our observations.

In our clinics we have noted that vestibular migraine is indeed much commoner than is duly recognised. We believe that it is an underrated and possibly underdiagnosed clinical cause of vertigo. It demands more awareness, better understanding and better appreciation. We are confident that if this unruly clinical condition is kept in mind in the forefront of memory and recall box, and not in the backyard, we may be able to avoid unnecessary and expensive vestibular tests, as indeed treat a larger number of patients more effectively. Stress and strain of life, racing against time and constant activity without any respite, aiming for higher goals, etc., are some factors that the modern life bestows upon us as an unwanted gift. We have reasons to believe that such and many other factors may contribute to the rising frequency of vestibular migraine.

In another study conducted by the same group (Neuhauser et al. 2005), it was observed that about 5 % of the population has vertigo at some point during the year and 7.4 % are affected at some point in their lives. They reiterated that vertigo is a frequent symptom in the general population with a 12-month prevalence of 5 % and an incidence of 1.4 % in adults. Its prevalence rises with age and is about two to three times higher in women than in men. The epidemiology of vertigo and underlying specific vestibular disorders is still an underdeveloped field despite its usefulness for clinical decision-making and its potential for improving patient care. The authors give an overview on the epidemiology of vertigo as a symptom and of four specific vestibular disorders: benign paroxysmal positional vertigo (BPPV), vestibular migraine, Meniere's disease and vestibular neuritis.

Another fine epidemiological research (Neuhauser 2007) is mentioned here for better appreciation of the incidence and prevalence of vertigo. This information can be used for clinical decision-making and help understand the underlying causes of vestibular diseases. The study pointed out that the diagnostic positional manoeuvres and treatments for benign paroxysmal positional vertigo, however, were still not being performed by most doctors. The female preponderance amongst patients with benign paroxysmal positional vertigo and migrainous vertigo was also noted. It may be linked to migraine but is not fully understood. The prevalence of Meniere's disease of 0.51 % was much higher than previous estimates. Follow-up studies had shown benign paroxysmal positional vertigo recurrence rates of 50 % at 5 years and a persistence of dizziness related to anxiety in almost a third of patients 1 year after vestibular neuritis.

Recent studies have underscored the impact of vertigo at the population level, but its effects and outcome on health and economy are not yet well known. Despite the fact that it brings about untold misery to a fairly significant portion of the population, it has not acquired due importance in life. Being a silent menace, it continues to remain dormant. Only those who suffer do realise the nuisance this debilitating clinical condition can bring into one's life.

Yet another study (Lempert and Neuhauser 2009) informs us that 1 year prevalence estimate for vertigo was 4.9 %, out of which 0.89 % had vestibular migraine and BPPV affected 1.6 %. The prevalence of Meniere's disease was 0.5 % higher than previous estimates by the same workers.

The impact of such a frequent problem on the economy of the nation and quality of life is another issue that has been partly dealt with in this book.

One study says that (Neuhauser and Lempert 2009) vertigo of vestibular or non-vestibular origin can both cause considerable impact on daily life. It is rated as one of the ten commonest causes of referral to a neurology clinic. In a German neuro-otological survey, vestibular vertigo accounted for 29 % of the cases seen by a doctor for vertigo. A recent Spanish survey (Garrigues et al. 2008) found that 0.8 % of the inhabitants in a primary care study consulted a primary care physician over 12 months for an illusion of unequivocal rotatory movement. The prevalence of primary care consultations for combined incident and recurrent dizziness was 1.8 % over 12 months in this Spanish study.

As a matter of fact, the neurology and the neuro-otology clinics deal with many more patients of vertigo than most other specialities. ENT is an exception, because vertigo is directly connected to the ears. No doubt the vestibular apparatus plays a significant role in maintenance of balance, but that is not the end of the story. Other bodily organs also have their own roles to play, which are equally important.

A detailed population-based survey carried out by Hain et al. (2011) in the USA showed that about 300,000 persons were affected by dizziness and vertigo between 1986 and 1988 per year. Approximately 26 % of them were unable to work. The authors calculated the economic loss brought about by the morbidity caused by vertigo to be approximately 2.25 billion $ each year.

According to this survey vestibular causes accounted for between 30 and 50 % of all cases of dizziness, followed by 5 and 30 % caused by medical conditions, between 2 and 30 % by neurological disorders, 15 and 50 % by the psychiatric disorders and at least 50 % remaining undiagnosed.

The following breakdown was given by the same author in a recent survey:
About 15 % of the population suffered with vertigo.
40 % due to otological reasons like labyrinthitis or CSOM.
10 % have central causes like an acoustic neuroma or multiple sclerosis.
25 % have medical conditions like the CVS diseases or drug induced.
25 % remain undiagnosed (idiopathic). Failure to establish the real cause.

Many patients of a certain age present in our clinics with a history of fall as the main presenting compliant. Some of them have genuine vertigo, others only light-headedness and unsteadiness. A detailed history must be taken to isolate a vestibular from other possible causes such as cardiovascular or metabolic diseases. Some patients may have diminished cerebral circulation due to age-related cerebral cortical atrophy and ischemic changes, which can be confirmed on a scan. Agarwal et al. (2009) also noted that balance disorders can be debilitating, sometimes leading to catastrophic outcomes such as falls. In their opinion the prevalence of vestibular dysfunction in the United States and the magnitude of the increased risk of falling associated with vestibular dysfunction had never been estimated. The prevalence of vertigo was therefore evaluated on the basis of some specific variables like the socio-demographics and the association between vestibular dysfunction and risk of falls.

This study demonstrated that between 2001 and 2004, 35.4 % of US adults aged 40 years and older had vestibular dysfunction. It was also noted that the odds of vestibular dysfunction increased significantly with age, which does not come as a surprise to anyone dealing with vertigo or dizziness on a daily basis. They also observed that the vertiginous symptoms were 40.3 % lower in individuals with more than a high school education and were 70.0 % higher amongst people with diabetes mellitus. It is hard to explain the former observation but not the latter. The study also mentioned that vestibular dysfunction with positive clinical symptoms had a 12-fold increase in the odds of falling.

We encounter the same problems in our clinics also. Many of our elderly patients would present with a history of repeated falls and head or bodily trauma. Sometimes they are confused even disorientated. Apart from an otological and vestibular assessment, they also require a neurological opinion. Many of such patients are then referred to the 'falls' clinic for further follow-up and management.

Their data showed the importance of diagnosing, treating and potentially screening for vestibular deficits to reduce the burden of fall-related injuries and sometimes deaths.

Numerous other studies have been carried out to establish the true extent of vertigo in different populations. Zingler and colleagues (2007) investigated the epidemiology of bilateral vestibulopathy (BV). They looked at over 250 patients with BPPV, diagnosed after a thorough investigation. They found out that 62 % of the cohorts had a past history of vertigo. The definite cause was determined in 24 % and the probable cause in 25 %. The most common causes found in their study were ototoxicity induced by aminoglycosides (13 %), Meniere's disease (7 %) and meningitis (5 %). Strikingly enough, 25 % of their patients exhibited cerebellar signs. As a matter of fact, cerebellar dysfunction was associated with peripheral polyneuropathy in 32 % compared with 18 % in vestibulopathy patients without cerebellar signs. Hearing loss occurred bilaterally in 25 % and unilaterally in 6 % of all patients. It appeared most often in patients with vestibulopathy caused by Cogan's syndrome, meningitis or Meniere's disease.

It is a very atypical study as ototoxicity is a relatively uncommon cause of vertigo in the UK. Meningitis likewise is an extremely rare condition. Besides, the volume of cerebellar signs reported in this study also appears to be far too high for a routine ENT clinic. These signs would be more often seen in a neurology clinic, which will make to study biased. The Cogan's syndrome, likewise, is an extremely rare condition and we have never encountered it in our practice.

We know that the disorders of balance are fairly common. But how common? Frankly there is no universal consensus on the actual figure. There is so much variation in the figures available in the global literature that one cannot be absolutely certain about the real frequency of this intractable malady that affects all ages. As a matter of fact, many of the so called 'idiopathic' causes reflect our inability to localise the cause, which obviously leads to the time-honoured need of further research.

Kroenke et al. (2000) carried out a Medline search and identified 12 articles containing original data on the aetiology of dizziness in consecutive patients. Dizziness was attributed to a peripheral vestibulopathy in 44 % of patients, a central vestibulopathy in 11 %, psychiatric causes in 16 %, other conditions in 26 % and idiopathic in 13 %. It was interesting to note that some of the serious causes were relatively uncommon, including cerebrovascular disease (6 %), cardiac arrhythmia (1.5 %) and brain tumour (<1 %).

Their conclusion was that dizziness was due to vestibular or psychiatric causes in more than 70 % of cases. Since serious treatable causes appeared uncommon, they believed that diagnostic testing could probably be reserved for a small subset of patients. We disagree with this study as most patients presenting in our department as surely in other ENT clinics are genuine cases of peripheral or central vestibular and not primarily psychiatric illnesses. The latter are referred by the family physicians to the relevant department and not an ENT clinic.

Generally speaking, the causes for vertigo are divided into two major categories, namely, the peripheral and the central causes. The common causes of peripheral vestibular vertigo are Meniere's disease, BPPV, vestibular migraine, labyrinthitis, vestibular neuronitis, ototoxicity, noise- and vibration-induced vestibular trauma, miscellaneous conditions, etc. The central causes include such conditions as acoustic neuroma, multiple sclerosis, cerebellar disorders or various CNS diseases. Some other causes of vertigo are of systemic origin: conditions like the cardiovascular diseases or diabetes.

There is a great deal of controversy in the classification of the causes of vertigo. Just as on its etiopathogenesis, Surenthiran (2001) laments that few studies have analysed the demographics of dizzy clinics and these have been limited by the numbers of patients studied or parameters analysed. Therefore, they looked at the case notes of patients attending their clinic for more than a decade. In this period, he noted that considerable socio-economic transition and medical advances had been observed without any significant change in the variables. Those with symptoms severe enough to warrant referral were relatively young and occupationally active. The spectrum of conditions diagnosed in the clinic demonstrated the important role of tertiary neuro-otology clinics.

One is obliged to agree with Surenthiran that such clinics are of immense value in managing the complex issue of balance with expertise. However, with the financial constraints and managed health care in full control, not all institutions or nations may be able to afford them.

One study (Hoshino et al. 1997, Hosch) involved a large number of patients attending such a clinic. It was noted that a high incidence of the patients in the fourth decade was noted, but the age distribution showed a recent tendency to shift towards older patients. The proportion of patients with peripheral vestibular disorders, diseases of the central nervous system, generalised diseases and others were 30.1, 17.7, 6.60 and 45.6 %, respectively. Meniere's disease was diagnosed in 6.67 % and BPPV in 4.72 % of all patients' viewpoint.

Many clinicians see vertiginous patients, and nearly each case presents a fresh dilemma.

Polenesek and colleagues (2008) looked at the vestibular disorders from a clinician's viewpoint; therefore, it interests us most. They believe that the vestibular impairment is an underlying cause in as many as 45 % of people complaining of dizziness. They agreed with the general observation that most causes of vestibular impairment can be effectively treated, but the diagnosis is often missed.

The aim of this study was to examine the clinical assessments used by health providers in evaluating dizzy patients in outpatient clinics and the emergency department. They employed computer-generated data for their study in which 157 patients were included. Over two-thirds of colleagues (69 %) used the patient's description of the dizziness for identifying the cause; however, they pointed out that a significant variability was evident across disciplines, ranging from 84 % of audiologists asking for a description of the dizziness to only 33 % in reply to the geriatricians. Interestingly enough 89 % of the colleagues dealing with the vertiginous patients did not evaluate their subjects for BPPV. It was also noted that primary care clinicians referred 22 % of dizzy patients to a specialist (neurotologist), while the geriatricians referred 17 %, and emergency physicians referred only 16 % of them.

The study duly highlighted the point that dizzy patients were not routinely screened for vestibular impairment based on available recommended practices, likely contributing to underdiagnosis and treatment. Their results indicated a need for effective dissemination of guidelines to improve health-care quality, increased awareness of medical risks and enhance patient access to appropriate treatment. And that certainly appears to be a valid plea, as many health-care facilities have little or limited information available to both staff and the patients. In an ENT clinic, you may find leaflets and booklets on anything from tonsillectomy to stapedotomy, but it is highly unlikely to find an information package, leaflet or literature on vertigo. It is badly needed, particularly for the elderly folks.

Ageing populations across the globe suffer with a variety of balance disorders. Not all of them have genuine vertigo. In our clinics we, specifically ask such probing questions as to determine whether they suffer from a rotational vertigo or simply feel unsteady on feet. Some may have BPPV, others simply a fear of fall due to loss of postural control. Many of the elderly folks have a history of bodily arthritis, knee or hip replacement surgery or just a stiff neck. These patients may actually have defective proprioceptive impulses travelling from the peripheral bodily parts, causing imbalance rather than a vestibular vertigo. The subject was studied in more than a thousand patients (Katsarkas 1994). In this study, 12.22 % patients were 70 years of age or older on the day of the first visit. In 39.13 % patients, paroxysmal positional vertigo was either confirmed or strongly suspected. In the 94.88 % confirmed cases, the observed paroxysmal nystagmus was compatible with excitation of the posterior semicircular canal. In 8.77 % patients, the dizziness could not be attributed to neurological or vestibular disease. Meniere's disease, vestibular neuronitis, vascular episodes and tumours were next in prevalence. The authors reached the conclusions that even though no difference was found in age distribution between women and men, dizziness was more prevalent amongst women.

Explaining the etiopathogenesis of disequilibrium in the elderly, they opined that the decline of behavioural and cognitive performances are due also to decline of biological rhythm control. The role of melatonin (the hormone regulating circadian rhythm) being strictly connected with cerebellar function was in question. It is a known fact that the cerebellum acts in elderly both at motor and cognitive regulation, which, according to this study, may be at fault.

They concluded that spatial orientation is altered in about 40 % of dizzy patients, but no significant differences were revealed in melatonin. It was worth noting that spatial memory was highly altered only in subjects with inversion of circadian melatonin rhythm. To explain it, they came up with a novel hypothesis that the alteration of the normal circadian melatonin rhythm played some role in the genesis of dizziness in a subpopulation of patients. Obviously further evaluation of this hypothesis would be required to confirm it. One must remember that imbalance in this age group may not fall under the category of vertigo *per se*, as they may not have rotational vertigo, a simple tendency to topple over. It may not be due to vestibular damage but due to other motosensory deficiencies such as defective locomotor system, diminished or altered proprioceptive impulses and exteroceptive impulses. Such deficiencies are not uncommon in the elderly. History and clinical examination should be able to confirm a clinical diagnosis. Vestibular investigations in such patients are usually not needed.

Further research into the role of melatonin in maintaining the circadian rhythm would be of immense interest to all those clinicians who have to deal with ageing populations. Furthermore, as hypothesised by these workers, more concrete proof is required to establish the association between the altered circadian rhythm and dizziness.

Older population anywhere in the world suffers with disorders of balance. The subject has been studied in many countries across the globe. Currently, Japan is struggling to meet the needs of its vastly ageing population. So is China. And that means a huge proportion of the world population indeed. Some workers investigated the association of disequilibrium with age (Weindruch et al. 1989).

The authors noted that in people aged 65 and older, disequilibrium is one of the most common diagnoses in short-stay hospitalisations, accounting for an average of 4.3 days of medical care. Older people without overt disease of any type tend to prove worse than the younger people. Considerable functional impairments may also add to the menace of imbalance. Deficits in postural control may be associated with an increased risk of falling. Other factors that may influence the geriatric disequilibrium may be vascular, visual, neuromuscular and pharmacological, each of which must be considered to understand and appropriately treat the disequilibrium.

The authors recommended that accurate identification of the cause of disequilibrium must involve the testing of multiple, interacting systems. The literature suggests that often no clear cause for an older person's disequilibrium can be found and indicates the possible existence of presently unappreciated etiologic factors. Progress in understanding these problems probably has been stymied by the fact that only a small, select subgroup of older patients are referred to specialists in otolaryngology. Quite probably, considerable progress on the understanding of the cause, diagnosis and treatment of geriatric disequilibria would result from more extensive research collaboration between otologists, geriatricians, epidemiologists and other specialists.

The ageing otolith membrane, alterations in calcium metabolism and ischemia have all been blamed as the possible factors. Senile deterioration of vestibular function on quantitative testing has been documented. Besides, senile cellular loss in the vestibular apparatus akin to a senile hearing loss is caused by the degeneration of the hair cells.

In the elderly population, a classical bout of vertigo may often be overshadowed by chronic or repetitive episodes of loss of postural control. As a matter of fact, a distinction may be made between the two through simple probing. Vestibular disorders in the older patients are riddled with problems like loss of independent activities, tendency to fall and overt or covert clinical depression. Co-morbidity is a contributor in many elderly. Some scientists are looking at the immunohistochemical expression of proteins in the basement membrane of the vestibular system in the elderly as a potential cause of the age-related decline in sensory cell and neuronal population. This subject has been discussed later in this book.

Loss of postural control is not the same as vertigo, because as we defined earlier on, a typical vertigo is 'a perception and not a reality'. On the contrary, the loss of balance in the elderly is a not a perception but a reality. There is a great deal of overlay between the two; hence, the exact frequency of one or the other can hardly be measured with certainty.

From several studies mentioned above, it becomes obvious that vertigo has many different aspects and each worker designs his study to look at yet another facet. One may however say with some assurance that the menace of vertigo is universal and involves all age groups, but it is a major contributor to burden of disease and disability in the adult population.

Another salient feature that emerges out of these studies is that the problem of vertigo is either misunderstood or underrated. Besides, many studies duly highlight the point that proper and timely referral from a family practitioner to a balance clinic makes matters a lot easier and simpler. Many cases of imbalance do not need expensive investigations like the VNG or an MRI scan. We are strong proponents of a clinical diagnosis, based upon a comprehensive and incisive history and a thorough clinical examination. Some cases however would require further evaluation at a dedicated vestibular lab. And some may remain undiagnosed despite all efforts. They fall into the category of 'idiopathic'.

The epidemiological studies mentioned here are mostly hospital based and therefore carry a bias. They only highlight the magnitude of problem, but more detailed prospective population-based studies are increasingly required to fathom the prevalence and the incidence of balance disorders. It should also be pointed out that despite all endeavours some cases of vertigo will remain etiologically undiagnosed. Such idiopathic cases demand further in-depth investigations.

Thus, summarising all these studies and our personal experience, it is submitted that the epidemiology of vertigo is still an underinvestigated field. Most studies are American or European. Many more regional studies are definitely required so that more appropriate and case-sensitive management could be planned.

For that and many other reasons, we are convinced that a routine ENT clinic dealing with a multitude of clinical conditions is not an ideal place for managing vertigo.

Ideally there should be an independent 'balance clinic' in each regional centre if not in every hospital. Hearing aids clinics are already being run by the audiologists quite successfully. Vertiginous patients on the same pattern may be referred by the family physicians directly to a balance clinic, which should be duly staffed by trained and qualified vestibular clinicians and scientists. Those failing direct referral criteria may be seen by an ENT specialist or a neurologist, depending upon the possible cause.

This practice is under trial in the British NHS at some major centres. Last year a pilot study was conducted in London, which duly underlines the benefits of this new concept. It was a UK hospital-based multidisciplinary balance clinic (Lee et al. 2011) run by allied health professionals. It was a retrospective review of the outcomes of nearly 200 patients.

The advantage was noted as the mean waiting time for the balance assessment clinic was 12 weeks (standard deviation 6 weeks). Furthermore, final decision regarding definitive management was made on the spot. Majority (74 %) of patients were referred for rehabilitation, 26 % required a review in the balance specialist clinic, 15 % underwent further investigations, 6 % were referred to the adult otology clinics and 1 required surgical intervention.

Obviously the burden of identification of vertiginous patients in a routine ENT clinic for definitive management can be significantly reduced through a dedicated balance clinic.

More significantly, the waiting time for vestibular rehabilitation was reduced from 21 to 15 weeks. They also note in this study that the patients were satisfied and no adverse outcomes were recorded.

This study opens new avenues for conducting a multidisciplinary balance clinic, run by allied health professionals. It certainly represents an alternative model for the management of patients with balance disorders. We feel that this is a way forward and should also be adopted by other centres dealing with vertigo.

References

Agrawal Y, Carey JP, Della Santina CC, Schubert MC, Minor LB (2009) Disorders of balance and vestibular function in US adults: data from the National Health and Nutrition Examination Survey, 2001–2004. Arch Intern Med 169(10):938–944, 0003–9926; 1538–3679

Committee on Hearing and Equilibrium (1995) Committee on Hearing and Equilibrium guidelines for the diagnosis and evaluation of therapy in Meniere's diseases. Otolaryngol Head Neck Surg 113(3):181–185

Garrigues HP, Andres C, Arbizar A et al (2008) Epidemiological aspects of vertigo in the general population of the autonomic region of Valencia, Spain. Acta Otolaryngol 128(1):43–47

Hain TC et al (2011) Epidemiology of dizziness. http://www.dizziness-and-balance.com/disorders/dizzy_epi_html. Accessed 12 Sept 2011

Hoshino I, Tokumasu K, Fujino A, Naganuma H, Arai M, Yoneda S (1997) Vertiginous patients seen at the neuro-otological clinic of Jitasato University Hospital during the past 25 years. Equilib Res 56(3):274–283, 0385–5716

Katsarkas A (1994) Dizziness in aging: a retrospective study of 1194 cases. Otolaryngol Head Neck Surg 110(3):296–301, 0194–5998; 0194–5998

Kroenke K, Hoffman RM, Einstadter D (2000) How common are various causes of dizziness? A critical review. South Med J 93(2):160–167, 0038–4348

Lee A, Jones G, Corcoran J, Premachandra P, Morrisona GA (2011) A UK hospital based multidisciplinary balance clinic run by allied health professionals: first year results. J Laryngol Otol 125:661–667

Lempert T, Neuhauser H (2009) Epidemiology of vertigo, migraine and vestibular. J Neurol 256(3):333–338, 0340–5354; 1432–1459

Neuhauser HK (2007) Epidemiology of vertigo. Curr Opin Neurol 20(1):40–46, 1350–7540

Neuhauser HK, Lempert T (2009) Vertigo: epidemiologic aspects. Semin Neurol 29(5):473–481

Neuhauser HK, Bon Brevern M, Radkhe A et al (2005) Epidemiology of vestibular vertigo: a neurotologic survey of the general population. Neurology 65(6):898–904

Neuhauser HK, von Brevern M, Radtke A, Lezius F, Feldmann M, Ziese T (2008) Burden of dizziness and vertigo in the community. Arch Intern Med 168(19):2118–2124

Polensek SH, Sterk CE, Tusa RJ (2008) Screening for vestibular disorders: a study of clinicians' compliance with recommended practices. Med Sci Monit 14(5):CR238–CR242, 1234–1010; 1643–375

Surenthiran SS (2001) General features and trends in patients presenting to a neuro-otology clinic. J Audiol Med 10(2):125–135, 0963–7133

Weindruch R, Korper SP, Hadley E (1989) The prevalence of dysequilibrium and related disorders in older persons. Ear Nose Throat J 68(12):925–929, 0145–5613; 0145–5613

Zingler VC, Cnyrim C, Jahn K, Weintz E, Fernbacher J, Frenzel C, Brandt T, Strupp M (2007) Causative factors and epidemiology of bilateral vestibulopathy in 255 patients. Ann Neurol 61(6):524–532, 0364–5134

Basic Sciences, Clinical Evaluation and Investigations

2

2.1 Posture and Balance

A clinician must fully understand the normal physiology of balance in order to identify a pathological factor. It has often been said that physiology is the mother of medicine and surgery. Its altered form is pathology. Therefore, we must fully comprehend the factors responsible for maintaining the posture and balance. Only then can we understand the factors that may be responsible for the dizziness that our patients may present with.

Balance is a complex physiological act involving a combination of factors. Appropriate information transmitted by the vestibular, ocular, exteroceptive and proprioceptive sensory receptors is gathered in the brainstem and the cerebellum, duly filtered out for necessary action. Any fault in this complex and intriguing setup may result in imbalance. Therefore, it may be safely said that a uniform and coordinated action of the CNS and peripheral sensory organs is responsible for the maintenance of posture and balance. The following systems control the balance.

1. Central nervous system
2. The ocular system
3. The vestibular system
4. The locomotor system

All animals are bestowed with four basic instincts, namely, hunger, security, curiosity and companionship. Mankind, probably more than the entire animal world. His quest for all these instincts to fulfil nay excel in, demands excellent bodily control. Posture and balance therefore play a huge role in the daily life of mankind.

Anthropologically and phylogenetically speaking, the fundamental difference between the animal kingdom and mankind is the attribute of intellect. In the words of Bergson, an eminent philosopher, the mankind possess intellect duly complimented with the faculties of reasoning and rationality, giving it superiority over other creatures.

Kant, another great philosopher, based his ethical theory of Deontology on the very principle of reasoning. It is a theory much liked by medical profession. It basically means that the 'means as well as the end' should both be good.

S.H. Zaidi, A. Sinha, *Vertigo*,
DOI 10.1007/978-3-642-36485-3_2, © Springer-Verlag Berlin Heidelberg 2013

Maintenance of posture and balance is a morphological process of evolution that has been granted to all living beings; however, the higher the status of the animal in the tree of evolution, the higher the state of standing posture. And balance does not simply mean the organised activity of physical form; reasoning also plays an important role in its maintenance.

It also includes the timely execution of an act, such as jumping off the cliff or diving into a cave. It is the higher faculty of reasoning and judgement that determines the final act. A decision to act or not to act is taken by the higher faculty; the job of the vestibulo-cerebellar complex is to obey the command of the master, i.e. the cerebral cortex. From the creepers and crawlers to the four-legged animals, it was a long jump indeed. But the evolution of Homo sapiens in itself was a giant leap into the future that happened several millennia ago. No wonder the contrast between the newborn of an animal such as a cow and mankind remains significant. The baby calf learns to stand on its feet maintaining its balance even though precariously, barely a few minutes after birth, whereas the human baby begins to hold its head after a few months and takes several more months to acquire a posture of standing upright; a posture that he learns to maintain and protect all along his life through the intricate system of vestibulo-oculo-cerebellar connections.

The vestibular system has an important role to play in the maintenance of balance. It does so in conjunction with the proprioceptive, exteroceptive impulses as well as the visual input transmitted through the vestibulo-ocular, vestibulo-spinal and vestibulo-collic reflexes.

The vestibulo-ocular reflex maintains a stabilised visual image on the retina during head rotation, by inducing compensatory eye movements. The vestibulo-spinal reflex stabilises the body in relation to gravity. The vestibulo-colic reflex is responsible for the stability of the head in space and acts specifically on the neck musculature. It also assists the vestibule-ocular reflex in stabilising visual activity. This reflex is also indicative of otolith function, specifically that of the saccule and is the origin of the term sacculo-colic reflex. The sacculo-colic reflex forms the basis of the vestibular-evoked myogenic potential. It will be discussed later on Mudduwa et al. (2010).

It is, however, the combination of several components that must act in harmony to achieve a desired effect. Akin to a symphony maestro conducting an orchestra, the cerebral cortex orchestrates the activity of all these components in a rhythmical, coordinated, articulated, predetermined fashion. Precision, economy of movement and discipline form the basic ingredients of an act of balance.

The vestibulo-cochlear element is deeply and rather safely sitting in the confines of the temporal bone.

The temporal bone has four components, namely, tympano-mastoid, the petrous, the squamous and the temporal. The vestibulo-cochlear component is located within the petrous bone. Standard textbooks of anatomy may be consulted for detailed description of the temporal bone, which is akin to a mother carrying the inner ear in its womb.

The inner ear is the main organ that is actually the hub of all activity related to the aural limb of factors controlling balance. The main components of the inner ear are the semicircular canals and the cochlea. There are two components within the semicircular canals, namely, the bony and the membranous labyrinths.

The bony part contains those elements that are essential for sensing the movement of body in relation to space. The semicircular canals are called the superior, posterior and lateral alias horizontal canals. They are located in a delicate and well-defined relationship with each other and with their contralateral counterparts so as to gather the information three dimensionally. The semicircular canals communicate with each other through a widened chamber called the vestibule. At the terminal end of each circular canal as it joins the vestibule, there is a slight expansion called the ampulla.

The superior or anterior canal gathers information about the movement approximately perpendicular to the temporal bone. The posterior canal gathers information from the direction of longitudinal axis of the temporal bone, and finally the lateral canal receives information from approximately the transverse bodily plane.

Since more details are beyond the scope of this book, the reader is advised for further reading to refer to an excellent description, in a chapter on anatomy and physiology by Seikel et al. or a similar standard book.

Each canal has approximately 90° angle between them and their orientation allows detection of angular acceleration in three planes.

The osseous labyrinthine capsule consists of two inner components. They are called the scala vestibuli and scala tympani. They are partly separated from each other by the osseous spiral lamina. As the labyrinth ascends from a wider base to reach the apex, scala vestibuli and scala tympani join each other at a very narrow point called the helicotrema.

The middle ear is separated delicately from the labyrinthine capsule by the round window, covered by a thin membranous structure called the secondary tympanic membrane, communicating the scala tympani with the hypotympanum. On the other hand, the oval window is covered by the footplate of stapes and isolates the scala vestibuli from the mesotympanum. In otosclerosis, which is really a metabolic disorder, the stapedial footplate is either perforated or removed partially or totally to bring the ossicular system in direct contact with the scala vestibuli by means of a prosthesis – stapedotomy (making a tiny hole in the footplate while retaining it) or stapedectomy (when the footplate of stapes is removed). Rarely the cochlea may be irreversibly damaged following this procedure. A perilymph leak following this procedure is an excepted outcome causing temporary vertigo, a sign of successful removal of stapes. Following the discovery of stapedectomy by Shea in the 1960s, which was allegedly accidental rather than intentional as the legend has it, the stapes surgery gained enormous popularity in the following three decades. It replaced the older procedures like fenestration for management of otosclerosis altogether. At least two generations of otologists performed stapes surgery with much relish, achieving dramatic results. Gradually the procedure has become less common as the crops of otosclerosis have been fully harvested. It is also perhaps due to decline in the prevalence of otosclerosis due to better dietary factors and quite likely the addition of sodium fluoride in the water supply. At one stage pioneering otologists like Schuchnecht advocated the consumption of sodium fluoride as a medical remedy for otosclerosis. It fell into disrepute partly due to the slow response to treatment and partly because the surgeons enjoyed doing stapedectomy with dramatic effects. It appears that sodium fluoride therapy may be returning back into limelight particularly for managing cochlear otosclerosis. The other obvious reason for the decline of stapedectomy or stapedotomy is the evolution of hearing aids from the clumsy body-held types to the fine behind-the-ear types (BTE) or the tiny 'in-the-canal types' which are barely visible.

Another important structure is the cochlear duct which communicates the labyrinth with the subarachnoid space of the posterior cranial fossa and hypothetically allows the drainage of perilymph contained within the bony labyrinth into the subarachnoid space. Perilymph has higher sodium content, almost like an extracellular fluid.

Within the bony labyrinthine capsule, the delicate and ultrasensitive membranous labyrinth sits rather snugly. It is constantly bathed in a highly refined fluid called the endolymph. The chemical composition of the endolymph is more like the intracellular fluid. The concentration of potassium which is so vital in maintaining the neural activity is relatively higher than in the perilymph. On the other hand, the sodium content is much lower than the perilymph.

The ampulla of each semicircular canal contains a delicate structure called the crista. It is a collection of highly specialised ciliated receptor cells along with a membrane. Over each crista rests a structure called cupula. Then there are the antennae-like structure called the sensory hair cells. The stereocilia or fine hairs are like a bunch of sensors checking out for a movement in a fluid medium and remain embedded within the cupula. There are two groups of hair cells called the outer and the inner hair cells and have different roles to perform. The outer hair cells tend to undergo physiological atrophy with age and are partly responsible for the functional loss. Currently much research is being carried out to replace the dying outer hair cells through eugenics. But one waits to see the results.

The macula of the utricle also has sensory hair cells or stereocilia covered with a fine jelly-like structure called the otolith membrane. It is gelatinous in texture and contains the sensory structures called the otoconia which are composed of calcium carbonate crystals and enable the inner ear to respond to gravitational changes called the otolith bodies. This fine dust of calcium carbonate, i.e. otoconia, remains suspended upon a matrix which sits on top of the hair cells. Since they are heavier in terms of specific gravity than the hair cells or the matrix itself, slightest of the otoconial movement exerts a shearing pressure on the hair cells. The hair cells bearing the responsibility of transmitting neurogenic information as the friction between the otoconia and their tips generates a series of neural fires.

As we shall see later on, the detachment of the otoconia is one common cause of vertigo. It is called the benign positional vertigo. The communication between the intracranial and the utricle–saccule compartments is maintained through a duct called the endolymphatic duct.

Suffice it to say that despite all the research there would always be a few cases that will remain undiagnosed aetiology wise and they fall under the category of idiopathic. It only reflects upon the deficiency in our understanding. More research is therefore the objective.

The actual organ of hearing is located in the organ of Corti. It has a very special role to perform in the transmission of the auditory signals. It is therefore securely placed within the tunnel of Corti and is bathed in an extremely specialised fluid, which differs chemically from both, i.e. the perilymph and the endolymph. It is the hair cells that are so very vital in the act of perception of sound signals that may be damaged due to several reasons; the commonest being the old age, leading to presbyacusis.

Once the hair cells perish, they cannot be recovered. But the new technologies involving the stem cell give us hope that sooner than later the damaged hair cells may be replaced. The same may also happen to the cochlea and the vestibular apparatus at some stage, one might hope!

2.2   Neurotransmitters

The role of neurotransmitters is duly highlighted in an excellent chapter written by Raymond et al. 1988. The reader is advised to read it to fully understand the types, forms and the composition of various neurotransmitters involved in maintenance of balance. In fact for a clinician this highly academic and research-based material becomes a bit complex to fully comprehend. We must, however, know the fundamentals to be able to translate the knowledge in clinical terms.

Six neurotransmitters have been identified that work between the three-neuron arc that drives the vestibulo-ocular reflex (VOR). Many others play a minor role. These neurotransmitters are glutamate, acetylcholine and GABA. Glutamate is responsible for maintaining the resting discharge of the central vestibular neurons and may modulate synaptic transmission in all three neurons of the VOR arc. Acetylcholine appears to function as an excitatory neurotransmitter in both the peripheral and central synapses. GABA is thought to be inhibitory for the commissures of the medial vestibular nucleus, the connections between the cerebellar Purkinje cells and the lateral vestibular nucleus, and the vertical VOR.

Three other neurotransmitters have a central mode of action. Dopamine may have a role to play in the all-important function of vestibular compensation. Norepinephrine may be responsible for modulating the intensity of central reactions to vestibular stimulation thus facilitating compensation. Finally the ubiquitous element histamine may have an all-important role to play. It is present centrally, but its role is not entirely clear. It is common knowledge that those antihistamines that work centrally modulate the symptoms of motion sickness (Crawford and Villis 1991).

Nausea and sickness are common companions of vertigo. There is an overlap in the biochemistry of motion sickness and vertigo. Acetylcholine, histamine and dopamine are the excitatory neurotransmitters that work centrally to control emesis. GABA is known to diminish the central emesis reflexes. Yet another important neurotransmitter serotonin is involved in central as well as peripheral control of emesis but has little influence on vertigo and motion sickness.

2.3   Vestibulo-Ocular Reflex

Affectionately called the VOR, it is a physiological action of the eyeball that is reflexive in character and is responsible for maintaining the images of objects on retina despite the movement of head in relation to space. It is responsible for producing the eye movement to the opposite direction of head movement thereby maintaining the image within the visual field. In many elderly folks noticeable and perceptible gentle head movement is a common observation, but in even young and healthy population, slight, almost imperceptible movement of head is present all the time. It is the function of the VOR to stabilise the image in subtle as well as obvious head movement so that a sharp image of the people and objects is maintained in the centre of the visual field. VOR does not stop functioning in neither darkness nor indeed when the eyes are closed.

VOR works in response to stimuli and signals received from the vestibular system. Since the primary role of the semicircular canals is to maintain balance through information provided about the horizontal movement of head in relation to space, the signals sent to VOR are rotational in nature. Those signals that originate in the utricle and the saccule, i.e. the otolith organs, send the signals for translational reflexes.

2.3.1   Translational VOR

The vestibular nuclei are responsible for generating the neuronic pathway for the rotational VOR. Head movement leads to the impulses that are generated ion semicircular canals, which are sent as signals through the vestibular nerve and Scarpa's ganglion, to terminate in the vestibular nuclei located in the brainstem. From the vestibular nuclei, new fibres emerge that cross over to the nucleus of contralateral abducens nerve. The sixth cranial nerve supplies and controls the movement of extraocular muscles. There are synapses with two other pathways. One carries information via the sixth cranial nerve to the lateral rectus muscle, a powerful extraocular mover of the eyeball. The other tract goes from the sixth cranial nerve by the abducens interneurons to the oculomotor or the third cranial nerve. These fibres control the activity of the eye muscles and mainly the medial rectus muscle, the powerful converger of the eyeball. Yet another pathway goes from the vestibular nucleus through the Dieters ascending tract to the ipsilateral medial rectus motor neuron, then there are inhibitory pathways from the vestibular nuclei to the abducens nucleus off the same side. Pathways for the vertical and tensional limb of the VOR are similar in nature and distribution.

There are some other direct pathways that drive and control the velocity of the ocular movement. Further details of all these intricate neural pathways can be obtained from the relevant literature and textbooks.

The whole act is fine tuned, coordinated and interdependent. In sideways movement of the head to the right, for instance, impulses are generated in the ipsilateral semicircular canals and sent ipsilaterally through the vestibular – Scarpa's – ganglion pathway. The impulses are immediately dispatched to the opposite abducens nerve, resulting in the stimulation of the lateral rectus of the opposite eye. Furthermore, by the action of the abducens internuclear interneurons and the third cranial nerve, the medial rectus of the same side is activated, thereby resulting in coordinate activity of both eyes leading to the drifting of the eye to the left, and vice versa.

A terminology used in vestibular testing is called the 'gain' of the VOR. It is defined as the change in the ocular angle divided by the change in the head angle during the head turn. Ideally the gain is 1.0. The gain of the horizontal and vertical VOR is usually close to one, but the gain of the translational VOR is generally low (Crawford and Villis 1991).

VOR can be assessed by the Halmagyi–Curthoys test. In this test the head is forcefully but carefully rotated to one side and controlled if the eyes succeed to remain looking in the same direction. When the vestibular system is disturbed a quick head movement to one side, no compensatory eye movement is generated, thereby resulting in the failure of the subject in fixating the gaze at a point in space. Same can also be performed through calorimetry, which is extremely reliable, but time-consuming and has few limitations, such as coronary artery disease.

In the CNS it is mainly the cerebral cortex that holds the commanding position. It is like a maestro conducting a symphony.

The cortex gathers all the information from various sources and acts upon the requisite information and the need to act. It sends its command through the lower motor neurons and the spinal cord for desired motor activity. It also informs the cerebellum of the action taken through the corticopontine-cerebellar tract. Constant feedback through the proprioceptive receptors and kinesthetic receptors also keeps the cerebellum continuously informed of the movements executed. The cerebellum is mainly responsible for transmitting the information received from the posterior columns and the spinal tracts to the cerebral cortex. Of the three components of the cerebellum, namely, archeo-, paleo- and neocrebellum, it is the neocerebellum that has the role of the chief of intelligence services, as a matter of speaking.

The cerebellum is so important in maintenance of posture that it deserves further description.

It is situated in the posterior cranial fossa and has dorsal relationship with the pons and medulla. The cerebellum has two hemispheres divided into lobes.

As mentioned before it has three components. Paleocerebellum sits anteriorly and receives proprioceptive information from the spinal cord. Its main function is to regulate posture through its control of antigravity musculature of the body.

The neocerebellum plays an important role in fine motor coordination and inhibits involuntary movements, possibly through the release of inhibitory neurotransmitters like GABA. Neocerebellum is indeed the most important component of the cerebellum. Not only does it process all the sensory information arriving from peripheral corners of the body but also applies breaks upon the unwanted, involuntary movements. It is the commonest clinical sign in the patients with cerebellar disorders, as they suffer with involuntary, unintentional tremors and digital movements.

The third part or the archeocerebellum is phylogenitically the oldest part of the cerebellum and maintains equilibrium.

The cerebellum carries out coordination of motor activity under the command of cerebral cortex to control the smooth movement such as that of muscles associated with the production of voice and speech. It does so through its connections with the pyramidal and extra pyramidal and the descending reticular formation.

The neocerebellum is particularly responsible for the sensory guidance of the higher centres in the execution of voluntary movements. It receives loads of information from the exteroceptive sensors of the bodily surfaces as well as the proprioceptive sensors in the muscles tendons and joints. It also receives all kinds of information from the ocular sources and the vestibular pathways. All that information is relevant for day-to-day life, but most of the information thus received may not be relevant at a particular time. Hence, some information has to receive priority over the other, and that is the main function of the neocerebellum.

For instance, if one is walking on a country path in semi-darkness, the eyes will transmit the factual information about the path as indeed of the ditch or a pot hole. It is the function of the neocerebellum to immediately filter out the information, withhold the information about the straight path and instantly release the warning to the cerebral cortex about the pot hole. It is then the job of the cerebral cortex to take an immediate action and instruct the locomotor system to act swiftly and escape an untoward fall into the ditch.

Cerebellar disease is associated with ataxia and dysmetria.

Maintaining balance under all conditions is an absolute requirement for humans, thus observed (Virk and McConville 2006). They agree with the general perception, indeed a reality, that maintenance of balance requires inputs from the vestibular, the visual, the proprioceptive and the somatosensory systems. How the CNS integrates all the inputs and makes cognitive decisions about balance strategies has been an area of interest for biomedical engineers for a long time. More interesting is the fact that in the absence of one or more cues, or when the input from one of the sensors is skewed, the CNS 'adapts' to the new environment and gives less weight to the conflicting inputs. The focus of this paper was a review of different strategies and models put forward by researchers to explain the integration of these sensory cues. Also, the paper compares the different approaches used by young and old adults in maintaining balance. Since with age the musculoskeletal, visual and vestibular system deteriorate, the older subjects have to compensate for these impaired sensory cues for postural stability. The paper also discusses the applications of virtual reality in rehabilitation programmes not only for balance in the elderly but also in occupational falls. Virtual reality has profound applications in the field of balance rehabilitation and training because of its relatively low cost. Studies will be conducted to evaluate the effectiveness of virtual reality training in modifying the head and eye movement strategies and determine the role of these responses in the maintenance of balance.

2.4   Past Pointing

The simple test of past pointing is a common finding in the cerebellar lesions. It means that a person intending to touch an object tends to overshoot. The cerebellum provides most of the motor signal that turns off a movement after it has begun. Therefore, if it is damaged or diseased, then the effective control of inhibitory activity would be compromised and the subject would not know when to check his movement. In clinical practice one employs this test on a daily basis by asking patient to shut his eyes and touch the clinicians index finger held at a central point in the line of his gaze. Alternating with his index finger of the right and then the left hand, he is asked to touch the physician's stretched out finger and then touch the tip of his nose. Normally one can do that without a problem, but if the patient has a cerebellar lesion, he may not touch the tip of his nose, instead overshoot towards either side.

2.4.1 Dysdiadokinesia

In response to a given command, the patient with normal cerebellar activity would raise and lower the arm in an orderly fashion. A patient with damaged cerebellum loses the perception of the instantaneous position of a part of body during a movement, resulting in disorderly, hasty and jumbled-up activities such as raising or lowering the arms. It is an extremely simple and clinical test that takes only a minute to check out the involvement of cerebellum as a possible cause of dizziness, indeed ataxia.

2.4.2 Dysarthria

It is the failure of appreciation of progression in a given act such as speech that requires rapid sequence of events like the command of the brain, laryngeal and oral activity motor in a coordinated manner. Lack of coordination between the various organs involved in neither production of speech nor indeed the appreciation of the intensity or the length of a given sentence makes a cerebellar patient stumble upon speech. He thus ends up in producing an incoherent and unintelligible speech.

Many patients with speech disorders are seen in our voice clinic and often enough referred to us for evaluation of the activity of the vocal cords with a nasoendoscopy. The patient may have suffered a stroke and may also have ataxia and altered speech. The vocal cords should be normal in these patients when asked to phonate or take a deep inspiration, confirmed on a stroboscopic evaluation. And yet they may have a defective speech, which may not be due to a lesion of the laryngeal breaches of the vagus but due to a higher lesion in the cerebellum. ENT physicians and surgeons should refer such patients to the speech and language team for further evaluation and management. The neurological opinion in such patients is obviously invaluable.

2.4.3 Intention Tremor

Normally if a patient is asked to touch an object sitting, he should do so in one smooth motion. A patient with cerebellar disease loses control over voluntary act of movement and first overshoots then moves his hand back and forth to reach the object.

2.4.4 Cerebellar Nystagmus

It is a movement of the eyeball that results from failure to fixate the eyeball on a spot which may be off centre. A rapid tremulous movement of the eye rather than a controlled gaze is another example of the failure of cerebellum to control the voluntary activity The information travelling from the vestibular organs go through the flocculonodular pathways and may be dysfunctional in a case of cerebellar nystagmus.

2.5   Hypotonia

Decreased tone of the peripheral musculature on the ipsilateral side is brought about by damage to the deep cerebellar nuclei. Diminished muscular tone is an important clinical sign of a cerebellar disorder.

The role of the vestibular system remains vital for maintenance of balance. Sudden change of the position of the head in relation to space as indeed the rapid movement, both fine and coarse needing adjustment of the body and torso to meet the demand of positional changes is managed through the semicircular canals. It will be discussed later on that the vestibular system is so delicate, so subtle and so swift that it sends the information to the sensory components of the CNS at a lightning speed for adapting instantly to the correcting posture of the body.

Cerebral cortex is like a commanding general, controlling its forces through an intelligence service, i.e. the sensory system for gathering information from far and wide and motor system for carrying out an action as and when required. Some of these actions, however, are voluntary such as moving an arm or a leg; others are involuntary such as the heartbeat.

Brain controls its subordinates through two pathways. They are (a) the pyramidal system and (b) the extrapyramidal system. The longitudinal tracts of the corticospinal system form the main pathways for the pyramidal system. The cortical cells send down long tracts through the medullary pyramid into the spinal cord and reaching the outermost peripheries through the distal pathways. These pathways are responsible for the control of delicate and fine movements so absolutely necessary for acquiring finer skills. The neural pathways, i.e. the axons and their masters in the cerebral cortex are called the upper motor neurons. Therefore, in clinical terminology those diseases that involve the corticospinal tracts and other upper motor neuron pathways are described as upper motor neuron diseases and can be singularly diagnosed by neurologists through detailed clinical survey.

The extrapyramidal tracts comprise of (1) the red nucleus, (2) substantia nigra, (3) subthalamic nucleus and (4) the brainstem reticular formation. The most important component of this system, however, is the basal ganglia, to which all these nuclei and tracts mentioned above are connected and are responsible for gross movements that cause required postural adjustments.

Both these systems, i.e. the pyramidal and the extrapyramidal, must function in conjunction and harmony to maintain balance.

The locomotor system comprises of the bones, cartilages, muscles, tendons, ligaments, joints and their arterial as well as the nerve supply. The anatomy of the locomotor system, as indeed its physiology, is extremely intricate and complex. The reader is referred to various standard textbooks on the subject. Suffice it to say though that the long and short bones, the long and brief muscles and the synovial and the non-synovial joints all form an essential part of maintenance of posture. The cranial nerves can in fact be traced down right up to the fines and the tiniest muscle or a joint in the body. No better example can be quoted here than that of the nerve to the stapedial muscle, a tiny muscle responsible for the important role of saving the cochlea from traumatic damage such as on exposure to a loud bang. It is supplied by a tiny branch arising from the facial nerve. In a case of traumatic facial paralysis, loss of stapedial reflex noted on checking for the middle ear reflexes can help localise the site of contraction or entrapment in a case of fracture of the temporal bone. By precisely localising the site of damage, an otologist can release the nerve in time and save the nerve from a state of neuropraxia to neurotmesis, even axonotmesis, showing a reaction of degeneration. Timely intervention in a traumatic facial nerve paralysis can save the patient a lifetime misery of an ungainly face. Ugo Fisch was one of the pioneering surgeons in the management of such cases. Some of us may have seen his surgical skills first hand. No one has been able to replace him, since he retired about a decade ago.

The long and powerful hamstrings and the calf muscles like the tibialis anterior and posterior or the intricate lumbricals or interossei all have a role to play in the maintenance of posture. Minute does not necessarily mean worthless. As a matter of fact, the finer positioning and manoeuvring of the feet is brought about by the humble interossei and lumbricals and not the mighty hamstrings.

The intricate network of the nerve supply to all these structures and the joints demonstrates the perfect way that nature has provided us with the control of our bodily posture. The long nerves supplying the muscles attached to the joint also supply the skin overlying the joint and the relevant muscles. Some of these fibres form the proprioceptive endings in the capsules of the joints and the attached ligaments. These endings are extremely sensitive to change of posture and any movement thus employed. They are connected through many sensory columns to the central nervous system which acts reflexly to command the motor arm of the locomotion system to respond swiftly to the need at the time.

Besides, from the body surfaces such as the soles of the feet or the back if sitting on chair or the bed in a supine stance, the exteroceptive impulses are dispatched through the posterior columns to continuously provide information about the texture, structure character, etc. of the surface in contact with the body. The righting reflex is a fine illustration of the way the body reacts if exposed to a sudden change of posture. For instance, if one is sitting on chair rolling and rocking back and forth and if he is suddenly pushed backwards rather forcibly or unexpectedly, the body responds by correcting the posture by immediately counteracting the motion through a forward jolt. Experimental physiologists often quote the example of a cat napping on her side. If something drops on her suddenly, she takes only a fraction of a moment to go straight into a jumping posture – an animal instinct of flight from danger!

Another example is that of a walk on a hard floor board in darkness. If the texture of the floor changes imperceptibly to a softer flooring such as a carpet, the exteroceptive and proprioceptive receptors will send the information to the higher centres to accommodate the posture according to the feel. But for a brief moment before all that takes place, one may tend to topple over even though for the tinniest of a moment. Surely most of us have experienced such a phenomenon on entering late in the cinema hall after the hall has been darkened!

Standing on a sandy beach is another example of the way the exteroceptive impulses modify the posture. As the wave comes in and washes away the sand from under the bare feet, the sudden change in texture makes one feel momentarily unsteady. These are all physiological actions and quite expected in a normal person.

Any pathology involving the exteroceptive, the proprioceptive or the righting reflexes will cause varying degrees of imbalance. A disease of not-so-distant past called syphilis used to affect the posterior columns in some untreated cases resulting in a condition called tabes dorsalis. The affected person failing to relay the relevant information from the floor to the higher centres would drag his foot or indeed lift and uncontrollably push it down onto the floor as he fails to do necessary adjustments in the distance between the floor and the lifted leg or appreciate the change of texture.

A person suffering a stroke or hemiplegia or paraplegia is another example where all other components of postural control are active except the systems that are faulty.

Then there are the vestibular nuclei. They also contribute through their tracts. The medial vestibulo-spinal tract contributes to the ascending and the descending portions of the medial longitudinal bundle. The ascending medial longitudinal fasciculus has connections with the extraocular muscles. Therefore, the medial longitudinal bundle in fact is responsible for organisation and execution of the cervico-oculo-vestibular reflexes; these reflexes in turn are essential in maintaining the coordinated eye–head movement.

The other important tract involved in maintenance of balance of course is the lateral vestibulo-spinal tract. It originates in the lateral vestibular nucleus which receives afferents not only from the eighth cranial nerve but also from parts of the cerebellum. The main function of the lateral vestibulo-spinal tract is the reflex spinal activity needed for the muscle tone.

The third tract having close connection with the vestibular nuclei is called the vestibulo-spinal tract. The fibres originate in the medullary and pontine reticular formation. They have strong inputs from the cerebellum, the accessory optic tract and the ascending spinal tracts. Apart from the control of respiratory and the circulatory system, experimental physiologists have shown that the stimulation of the reticular system influences the muscle tone and facilitate or inhibit the activity generated in response to the pyramidal system and the reflex activities called the mitotic reflexes.

In order to fully understand the principles of management of the dizzy patient, it is absolutely essential that one has the firm knowledge of the factors that control balance. It is the fault in any of these controlling factors or a combination of them that may cause vertigo.

Physiological giddiness is a normal response which must be fully differentiated from a pathological dizziness. For instance, it is expected of a normal person to feel momentarily dizzy on looking down to earth from a certain height, say the top of the Empire State building or the Eiffel Tower, but is quite another matter for someone to feel extremely giddy even sick and unwell at lesser heights. One is a normal phenomenon, the other an exaggerated vestibulo-ocular response. It is also called acrophobia.

Two cranial nerves are extremely important from the viewpoint of a physician dealing with vertigo. That does not exclude the need for knowing about the other remaining cranial nerves, but from day-to-day relevance point of view, the oculomotor nerve and the vestibulocochlear nerve are more important. Therefore, knowledge about their nuclei and pathways is essential.

The oculomotor or the third cranial nerve has two components. It carries general somatic impulses from all the ipsilateral extrinsic ocular muscles through an efferent pathway except the superior oblique and lateral rectus. The third cranial nerve nuclei are located in the midbrain. The fibres from the nuclei carry impulses through the red nucleus emerging to form an inferior and a superior branch to supply the muscles that control inwards, upwards, downwards and laterally.

The general visceral efferent fibres beginning in the Edinger–Westphal nucleus are responsible for perception of light and controlling accommodation through papillary control and coarse as well as fine focus onto the objects.

The vestibulocochlear nerve is the nerve of hearing and balance. Since hearing goes parri passu with hearing in a normal child, it therefore has not two but three important roles. Its special somatic afferent component transmits information regarding hearing and balance. The efferent component on the other hand seems to help in the selective damping output of hair cells.

The vestibular nerve has two divisions, namely, the superior vestibular nerve and the inferior vestibular nerve. The former supplies the lateral and superior semicircular canals and the latter innervates the posterior semicircular canal and major part of the saccule.

The acoustic branch gathers information generated at the cochlear level and transmits it to the spiral ganglion located inside the modulus of the osseous otic capsule. The spiral ganglion consists of the bodies of the bipolar cells projecting their axons through the internal acoustic meatus. These fibres then join the vestibular nerve fibres and enter the medulla oblongata close to the pons to synapse with two important nuclei, namely, the dorsal cochlear and the ventral cochlear nucleus.

The second component of the eighth cranial nerve, namely, the vestibular nerve, relays the information about the acceleration and location in relation to space to the vestibular ganglion situated inside the internal auditory meatus. Fibres reach the pons and medulla and synapse with the superior, inferior, medial and lateral vestibular nuclei. These nuclei project to the spinal cord, thalamus, cerebellum and the cerebral cortex, thus establishing the pathway for the maintenance of balance.

The auditory nerve is not discussed here in detail but involves a concentrated effort of a combination of olivo-cochlear bundle, the medial and lateral superior olives, the medial geniculate body and the auditory radiations, projecting from the medial geniculate body into the Herschel's gyrus also called the area 41 of the temporal bone. It is located in close proximity to area 42 which is an auditory association area that communicates with other parts of the cortex and also to the opposite auditory cortex through corpus callosum.

The reader is referred to standard textbooks of anatomy and physiology for more detailed reading.

There are numerous clinical conditions that can cause vertigo. Some of the salient amongst them are Meniere's disease, benign positional vertigo, vestibular migraine, vestibular neuronitis, viral labyrinthitis, cervical vertigo, age-related vertigo, ototoxic vertigo, noise-induced vertigo and many cardiovascular and metabolic conditions. There are a few central causes which are discussed here such as acoustic neuroma and multiple sclerosis. Many other causes may have to be dealt by other relevant specialities and are beyond the scope of this book. And yet there are many cases where we cannot establish the cause. They are labelled as 'idiopathic'.

2.6   History and Clinical Examination

It is essential that a detailed history must be taken prior to conducting a thorough clinical and physical examination. Of course in some cases further investigations would be inevitable such as the vestibular function tests or imaging. But in most situations the diagnosis is clinical.

The history must begin at the beginning. Just like any other clinical condition, detailed interrogation and listening to the patient without interruption are absolutely vital. The physician who has the patience to pay total and undivided attention to the patient's narration of his symptoms is the one who reaps the rich harvest of success at the end of an interview. Listening rather than talking is always the best practice, often applied by many seasoned physicians.

Details of the presenting complaint and its mode of onset; length and duration; intensity; associated symptoms, such as tinnitus, hearing loss, nausea, sickness, tendency to fall, headaches, migraine, palpitation, syncope and fainting attacks; drugs; and any other systemic or metabolic condition such as a heart or coronary artery diseases, diabetes and epilepsy must all be recorded. These are some of the pieces of the jigsaw puzzle and form an essential part of a proper history.

Several illustrations of our history taking are described in the relevant case reports. The commonest questions that are asked are tabulated here as a questionnaire.

2.6.1   Questionnaire

Description of the present episode.
Room spinning, objects moving around, the whole world going upside down.
Duration. How long did it last?
Were you confined to bed?
If so, for how long?
Did the dizziness come with rolling over in bed or attempting to get out of the bed?

Was it initiated or aggravated by looking up or down or picking an object from the floor or the ceiling?

Any other symptoms (particularly tinnitus, fullness of the ears or hearing loss).

Nausea, sickness and vomiting.

Headaches, migraine, photophobia, oscillopsia and any form of aura.

Sweating and pallor.

Tendency to fall over.

Fainting and collapse.

Can you walk without support?

Any heart condition, light-headedness and stroke.

Diabetes.

Ear infections, discharge and surgical treatment if any.

Any other illness, e.g. epilepsy, tremors, disturbed gait. Veering to either side on walking.

Vision. Any eye condition, glaucoma, limited peripheral vision and macular degeneration.

Arthritis and neck stiffness. Shoulder and backache.

History of a joint replacement surgery.

Drugs and medication.

Past history of similar episodes, duration and treatment.

Any history of family illness of a similar nature.

Any neurological illness or deficits.

Anxiety, depression, emotional trauma and phobias.

Hyperventilation or panic attacks.

Psychiatric illnesses.

Any other relevant information.

As a fundamental rule, one should avoid asking direct questions; however, sometimes it may be necessary to prompt a thought process by obliquely asking about relevant symptom. Much too often as an experienced physician may vouch, the elderly patients seem to drift away from the point of focus. So more like a correcting device, one may ask a relevant direct question. By and large, however, the patient must be allowed, indeed encouraged, to give detailed account of the symptoms of dizziness. Remember a true vertigo is located in the senses. It may be described in many ways, such as things and objects moving, revolving, rotating or going upside down. It is all about perception and description of the events. Communication skills of individuals vary from poor to excellent.

It is particularly important to concentrate on the history of headaches, photophobias, phonophobias or any other forms of aura. Migraine is an essential cause of dizziness and is underrated. Tinnitus is more common than people seem to think. It is an extremely distressing and rather difficult condition to cope with.

Akin to vertigo, tinnitus is also a sensual symptom. Such noises as described by the patient as 'in the ear' or 'inside the head' are purely subjective and are obviously not present in the surroundings. We must, however, mention that an odd case of objective tinnitus was seen by one of the authors many, many years ago. It could be caused by overactive stapedial or the tensor tympani, reacting rather aggressively to an audible sound akin to a myoclonus. But that is an exception rather than a rule. Most cases of tinnitus with vertigo are subjective, varying in pitch, intensity, duration, forms and degree of nuisance. Otosclerosis is a known cause of tinnitus. But other than that, in most cases a specific cause cannot be established. It can be a ringing sound or a hissing sound and a buzzing in the head or complete musical tunes almost like the sound of a recognisable music instrument. It has been described as musical imagery tinnitus. Sometimes such patients are wrongly referred to a psychiatry department, supposedly suffering with hallucinations. Some patient may indeed have a history of grief, tension, stress and anxiety. A few may actually have a known mental illness.

Much reassurance during discussion on its management is needed, as most of the times we cannot eradicate it. Its attribute like intensity and variation of tone, whether unilateral or bilateral, must all be recorded. Frankly without digressing from the subject, one hastens to add that more research and efforts must be put on the subject of tinnitus. It is a very depressing, indeed troublesome, condition with little available in terms of help except a tinnitus masker.

One must never forget the importance of hearing loss in the matters of vertigo. Many times, imbalance and hearing impairment go hand in hand. The hearing deficit may not be an isolated accompaniment of vertigo; tinnitus is an important symptom that often troubles such patients too.

There are numerous clinical conditions that one has to ponder over as the detailed history is taken. Once a thought process starts the clinical mind normally starts to eliminate many things concentrating over those that seem to be relevant in a particular situation. One must never, however, switch off the thought process as many false traps remain hidden in the bushland of clinical dilemmas, so often encountered in the management of vertigo.

History taking may be exhaustive, but depending upon the physician's experience, it may take only a few minutes to pinpoint the problem and concentrate on the most probable cause. To sift through a lot of information and arrive at a conclusion is an art that matures with age and experience. Sometimes it is akin to searching for a needle in a haystack! But it is highly rewarding.

Thabet (2008) discussed the importance of detailed and precise history taking and avoidance of unnecessary and expensive investigations, in an article. They looked at the feasibility of differentiating the cause of acute vestibular syndrome in vertiginous patients using clinical, audio-vestibular and radiological tools. They performed a case series for study of patients complaining of acute vertigo at a university referring centre for hearing and vertigo. In this study, 30 patients with a history of acute vertigo without any history of previous otological or neurological disorders were evaluated. Eighteen of them were found to be due to an acute peripheral vestibular lesion, 1 had a psychiatric problem and was on antidepressant drugs, but interestingly enough 11 had a central vestibular lesion. One would presume that these patients would have undergone further investigations and perhaps imaging as well as neurological opinion.

Thabet (2008) identified these causes on precise and detailed history taking. They concurred with other clinician's observation and daily practice that the most important step in the diagnosis of acute vertigo is a thorough and detailed history. The common error of carrying out investigations instead is to be avoided. The clinical evaluation has the highest sensitivity and specificity in differentiating central from peripheral vestibular lesions.

Following the history, the clinical examination should take only a few more minutes in a clinical setup. The examination begins with simple observations like the overall condition of the patient, his physical form, his demeanour, his expressions, his gait and any telltale signs that might help in arriving at a diagnosis.

The clinical examination begins with the examination of the face for any asymmetry, as the facial nerve palsy may be associated with vertigo such as in Ramsay Hunt syndrome. Also the telltale signs of an attack of viral infection, e.g. herpes with vesicles around the pinna and in the upper part of the neck, which may be quite painful in Ramsay Haunt syndrome or in herpes zoster oticus or shingles, less so in other non-specific viral exanthemata.

The ears should be examined for any congenital or acquired lesions. Inspection of the pinna, the mastoid region, the ear canal and the tympanic membrane should follow. Surgical scars should be noted and investigated. A pre-auricular sinus is not an unusual finding. If symptomless, it may be left untouched, albeit noted down.

It should be followed by an examination with an otoscope, viewing the external auditory canal for any signs of inflammation, pus discharge, secretions, swelling or a mass. The colour of discharge and associated tenderness may be relevant. For instance, the fungal infection called otomycosis is a painful acute condition of the outer ear with either whitish discharge caused by Candida albicans or more likely black, indicative of Aspergillus niger.

A boil in the ear is an extremely painful condition and an otoscope may not be introduced in the outer ear without warning the patient about ensuing pain. The pinna may be protruded forward and the post-aural sulcus may be obliterated in more severe acute external ear infections. The eardrum must be examined thoroughly looking at the colour which should be pearly white; the pars flaccida and pars tensa, the two components of the eardrum; the position of the handle of malleus, which should be vertical, but the umbo should be just a wee bit behind the midline; the cone of light, which is always the antero-inferior position on each side; and finally the mobility of the eardrum on performing Valsalva's manoeuvre which should be positive, i.e. resulting in outward mobility of the eardrum in normally functioning ear and the Eustachian tube.

If the drum is pinkish, or congested, one may be dealing with an acute middle ear infection. If it is dull and retracted, then there might be a fluid in the middle ear. Sometimes one may be able to see a hairline or air bubbles supporting the diagnosis of a so-called glue ear. If the drum is featureless without a discernible cone of light and faded colour, failing to move with a pneumatic speculum or on Valsalva's manoeuvre, it may be due to a Eustachian dysfunction, and finally if the drum is blue, it may be an indication of serous effusion in the middle ear, though an extremely rare condition, a chemodectoma of the superior jugular bulb arising from the floor of the middle ear when the floor may be dehiscent. It is a significant condition to keep in mind. It produces an effect described as the 'rising sun appearance' due to the silhouette produced by the movement of the drum with a pneumatic speculum against a back drop of the bluish chemodectoma. A pulsatile unilateral tinnitus or a unilateral conductive hearing loss may be the only symptoms in such as a case.

Signs of otitis media, namely, capillary injection, congestion, inflammation, perforation, discharge, bleeding, a polyp or the presence of granulation tissue, must all be noted down. Ideally as an otologist should examine the ear under a microscope as any experienced clinician may uphold the statement that some atrophied eardrums may indeed mimic an atelectatic drum or a healed perforation. Such eardrums may indeed be thin and nearly useless functionally, in terms of mobility and transduction of sound, albeit of some use, if tightly plastered to the ossicles resulting in a columella effect as in myringo-stapediopexy. A common observation in any ENT clinic is to see a case of tympanosclerosis. It is sometimes called an adhesive otitis media. Basically it means that the middle ear infection has settled down and the telltale signs of a whitish, discoloured, lustreless and featureless drum remain only as the relics of the past. The chalky deposits could be confined to the drum only, when it is called myringosclerosis, or involve the ossicles and the promontory as well, when it is called tympanosclerosis. Vertigo is an unusual symptom in these cases but hearing impairment is nearly always present. It may vary in intensity from mild to severe depending upon the degree of the sclerotic patch. Some patients who may have had a myringotomy with grommet alias ventilation tube insertion in the past may also present with myringosclerosis.

One important test in the otological examination which has somewhat receded into background is called the fistula test. It should always be performed in cases of labyrinthitis caused by cholesteatoma, as indeed in perilymph fistula. It involves either using a pneumatic speculum or simply increasing and releasing the pressure manually in the external auditory canal to elicit vertigo while looking for horizontal nystagmus. If positive the test almost always indicates a labyrinthine involvement, such as erosion caused by chronic suppurative otitis media. It has also been described as the Hennebert's sign.

The cranial nerves play an important role in defining the causes of vertigo. It is left up to the neurologists to carry out detailed neurological evaluation, but an otolaryngologist must perform a thorough checkup of the cranial nerves in a case of a dizzy patient. The cranial nerves that matter most, of course, are the vestibulocochlear nerve, the facial nerve, the trigeminal nerve and the oculomotor nerve. But other cranial nerves should not be forgotten. The detailed evaluation of the cranial nerves, including the assessment of their motor, secretomotor or sensory functions, is described in standard clinical textbooks.

Every medical student has to learn the art of neurological evaluation during his clinical posting in medicine. One cannot overemphasise the importance of hands on problem solving method of learning in the medical profession.

Besides, since the cranial nerves are not the only relevant components, one should never forget the role of spinal tracts in transmitting both sensory and motor impulses across the peripheral parts of the human body.

In a busy clinical practice, it is not always possible to carry out a detailed neurological examination of each dizzy patient, but some salient observations and physical examinations must never be compromised.

2.6.2   Basic Clinical Examination

Examination of the ear, with an otoscope or under the microscope.
Look for nystagmus.
Past pointing and finger-to-nose test.
Tremors, intentional or non-intentional and fine or coarse.
Cranial nerve examination.
Ataxia and dysarthria.
Gait and postural control.
Unterberger's test.
Romberg's test.
Head thrust.
Dix–Hallpike test.
Audiometry.

Amongst the many salient features, nystagmus plays a singularly important diagnostic role. Volumes of literature are available for an interested person to read through in standard textbooks. From a clinician's point of view, suffice it to say that we look for horizontal nystagmus in most peripheral cases of vertigo and vertical or rotatory nystagmus in suspected central causes.

Horizontal nystagmus has two components, often described by the physiologists as the slow phase and the fast phase. The slow phase involves the drifting way of the eyeball laterally in very gentle sometimes imperceptible movement. It is the natural outcome of the underlying pathology. The fast component of nystagmus is inward or medial rapid movement of the eyeball as if in haste to bring the eye back to its resting position. The slow phase is brought about by the vestibulo-ocular reflex and the fast component is the outcome of the compensatory forces that do not wish the eye to drift way laterally.

The direction of nystagmus is a good clinical indicator of the side of vestibular pathology, in horizontal or so-called peripheral nystagmus. It should be the direction of the slow phase that should determine the direction of nystagmus; however, since this component is usually too subtle and can often be missed out, by convention the physiologists have taught us to look for the rapid component of nystagmic beat, which is obviously easy to pick out, and describe it as the direction of nystagmus. Therefore, by the process of logical interpretation, then the slow phase has to be to the opposite side and the side of pathology.

Its importance lies in the fact that by identifying the direction of nystagmus, one can identify the involved labyrinth, as most peripheral pathologies would cause the nystagmus to beat away from the side of the lesion. For instance, if the nystagmus is directed to the right, one would look for the cause in the left labyrinth, and vice versa.

The second important indicator in observing for nystagmus is the degree of nystagmus.

Three degrees have been described for the nystagmic beats. The first degree nystagmus means that the eye beats faster on looking towards the direction of nystagmus, i.e. the fast component (Alexander's law). So, for instance, if the nystagmus is directed to the right, i.e. the fast component is towards the right, then in the first degree nystagmus, the eye beat becomes more pronounce on asking the patient to look towards right. The first degree nystagmus is an indicator of relatively mild pathology in the vestibular apparatus.

The second degree nystagmus is the one that continues to beat albeit with preponderance towards the direction of the fast component when the patient is asked to look straight on. It indicates a somewhat more significant underlying cause in the vestibular system. It also implies that despite the forced discourage net of the ocular system, the vestibulo-ocular reflex is potent enough to counteract the inhibiting effect.

The third degree nystagmus means that when asked to look in the opposite direction of the nystagmus, the eye beat continues to persist though somewhat reluctantly. It underlines the possibility of a more intense degree of vestibular disease (Dell'Osso and Daroff 1999).

From the practical point of view, the lesion in vestibular nystagmus lies in the end organ, nerve or brainstem. Calorimetry is a fine example of normal activity of the vestibular end organ on deliberate stimulation with warm or cold water or nowadays the use of air. The nystagmus beat is directed to the opposite side with cold stimulant and to the same side with warm stimulant. It was made easier for us in the early part of training to recall it as a mnemonic HS:CO (house surgeon: casualty officer). It is also expected of a normal subject to experience dizziness which may vary in intensity and sometimes may result in retching and vomiting. The test may have to be abandoned in some situations. Besides, a normal subject is expected to past point and fall in consistent direction on performing the Romberg's test. The important thing to remember is that pass pointing and Romberg's are always in the direction of the slow phase. The effects of a cold stimulant mimic a destructive lesion of the vestibular end organ as seen in post-labyrinthectomy cases of intractable vertigo. In unilateral Meniere's disease, the nystagmic beat may be ipsilateral.

Many years ago some ENT physicians used to employ single stimulus of ice cold water in a very tiny amount. It would excite the labyrinth intensely and an observation was made by noting the nystagmus and its duration. It was called the Linthicum test. It never gained popularity as it was much too intense a stimulus and the patients often felt very unwell afterwards.

It is worth remembering that a patient with unidirectional jerk nystagmus, feeling of dizziness at looking in the direction of the fast phase, with past pointing and positive Romberg, in the direction of the slow component may have a peripheral vestibular disorder of the end organ to which the slow phase is beating (Dell'Osso and Daroff 1999).

It is a simple but extremely useful clinical tip for a practitioner to keep at the back of his mind while examining a patient suspected to have a peripheral vestibular lesion.

It is the slow phase that displays the side of the lesion, but can be missed out due to its faintness. The fast component of nystagmus is easy to pick up. So by a process of elimination and mental calculation, the pathological side is presumed to be on the side of the slow phase.

Whenever the pattern of the direction of nystagmus, vertigo, past pointing and Romberg fall is not as just described but varies in some aspect, the symptom complex may represent an abnormality of the central vestibular nuclei. In such a situation, the vertigo may be felt looking in the direction of the slow phase of the nystagmus, and the past pointing or Romberg fall may be towards the fast phase (Dell'Osso and Daroff 1999).

It is a general teaching that a slow phase usually represents the side of peripheral vestibular pathology but may also represent ipsilateral central cause.

Acoustic neuroma may show a horizontal beat, which is contralateral to the side of the lesion, particularly if fixation is eliminated. A combination of a small amplitude rapid primary position jerk nystagmus beating contralateral to the lesion and a slower larger amplitude gaze-evoked (Burns') nystagmus ipsilateral to the lesion also occurs with extra-axial masses including cerebellar tumours, compressing the brainstem (rarely Burns') nystagmus is inverted (Yokota et al. 1993).

This is an extremely useful tip for a practitioner yet again. Simple observation and very basis tests like the Romberg's test can lead the physician onto the right path.

In fact we have encountered a few cases of arachnoid cysts in our practice, diagnosed radiologically in our vestibular clinic. They simply need a regular follow-up, usually by the neurologists. These patients were suspected to have a central lesion on clinical observation, duly confirmed by imaging.

Vertical or rotatory nystagmus is seen infrequently in an ENT practice. It is usually an almost certain sign of a central pathology. Neurologists see this form of nystagmus in their practices more often than we do.

Since vertigo is a subjective condition and cannot be seen by the onlooker unlike say a rash or a boil or an abscess, its salient as indeed silent clinical sign is the nystagmus. Since it is a major indicator of an underlying clinical condition, it must be evaluated with some considerable deliberation. Many times the nystagmus beat is too soft to be picked up; hence, a magnifying device like the Frenzel's lens may be employed for gaining a clear view of the eye movement. In day-to-day practice, however, it is seldom used in a routine otolaryngological outpatient department.

One particular type of nystagmus that may sometimes be confused with a serious pathology is a congenital condition called the miners' nystagmus. In certain developmental errors of the eye mainly retina, the eye seems to flicker about horizontally with a brisk speed. It may be seen in albinos too, but more often in conditions like the Marcus Gunn phenomenon, where the eye tends to twitch unduly due to an aberrant branch of abducens nerve and displays rather fine sometimes coarse nystagmus. The whole point being that the intraocular muscles perpetually attempt to bring the eye to apposition where the image could fall on the fovea in retina.

The congenital nystagmus is wrongly called the miners' nystagmus on account of the miners spending much time underground, only to emerge in the light to struggle to focus. It is obviously a misnomer.

Such a nystagmus has no bearing on the vestibular apparatus and one must be cautious in determining the nature of congenital nystagmus in a busy clinical setup and not create undue panic by ordering multitude of expensive investigation. In these days of austerity, rising cost and rationing of services, one must be prudent enough to select the cases in need of detailed investigations such as the MRI or vestibulometry.

Congenital nystagmus is usually present at birth and persists throughout life. It is quite easy to pick up and diagnose through history and simple clinical observation. It is binocular with equal amplitude and can be provoked or at least increased by an attempt to fixate the eye at an object. It is usually modulated by gaze and not evoked by it. More interestingly, it diminishes with a constant gaze or convergence.

Most common presentation of a congenital nystagmus is that it is horizontal and rarely vertical. It has many other attributes, which are best picked up by an ophthalmologist or a neurologist. From an ENT point of view, the fundamental fact that a nystagmus which is congenital is self-evident in history taking is sufficient enough to avoid unnecessary vestibular tests. Most such patients would have been to see an ophthalmologist before visiting us.

Dizziness remains one of the most common reasons for which the patients visit their physicians (Yokota et al. 1993). It was reminded in this study that the control of balance depends on receiving afferent sensory information from several sensory systems, vestibular, optical and proprioceptive, exteroceptive, etc. Bioelectric signals, generated by body movements in the semicircular canals and in the otolithic apparatus, are transported via the vestibular nerve to the vestibular nuclei. All four vestibular nuclei, located bilaterally in medial longitudinal fasciculus, are linked with central nervous system structures. These central nervous system structures are involved in maintaining visual stability, spatial orientation and balance control. Nystagmus is a result of afferent signal balance disorders.

The author opines that the nystagmus due to peripheral lesions is conjugate nystagmus, because there is a bilateral central connection. Lesions above the vestibular nuclei induce deficits in synchronisation and conjugation of eye movements; thus, the nystagmus is dissociated. This paper shows that in peripheral vestibular disorders spontaneous nystagmus is rhythmic, associated, horizontal-rotatory or horizontal, with subjective sensation of dizziness which decreases with time and harmonic signs whose direction coincides with the slow phase of nystagmus, and it is associated with mild disorders during pendular stimulation with statistically significant vestibular hypofunction. Spontaneous nystagmus in central vestibular lesions is severe, dissociated, horizontal, rotatory or vertical, without changes related to optical suppression; if vestibular symptoms are present, they are nonharmonic.

In central disorders, findings after thermal stimulation with cold or warm water or air are either normal or pathological, with dysrhythmias and inhibition in pendular stimulation. This paper also deals with differential diagnosis of vertigo based on anamnesis and clinical examination, as well as objective diagnostic tests.

The reader is referred to an excellent write-up on further details of nystagmus and for in-depth understanding of the nuances of saccades and oscillations in nystagmus (Dell'Osso and Daroff 1999).

2.7   Head Impulse Test

In search for an easy bedside or simply clinical diagnostic tool, the head impulse test is gaining popularity.

As described elsewhere in this book, this test is an important tool, particularly in the diagnosis of acute problems such as vestibulitis (Paine 2005). One important role of this test is to differentiate between acute vestibular neuritis and cerebellar infarction. In patients with acute vertigo but abnormal head impulse test, acute vestibulopathy is ruled out and cerebrovascular causes such as brain ischaemia even an infarct should be considered (Sloane et al. 1989). Normally the vestibular system rapidly adjusts to the slightest of the change of the position of head so that the centre of vision remains within a clear view. In a case of vestibulitis, if the head is turned towards the involved side, a delay is noticed as the momentary fixed gaze towards the ipsilateral side is instantly followed by a corrective saccadic movement of the eye in an effort to bring it back to the centre.

McGarvie and Halmagyi (2009) designed a study to develop an easy-to-use video HIT system (vHIT) as a clinical tool for identifying peripheral vestibular deficits. They also wanted to validate the diagnostic accuracy of vHIT by simultaneous measures with video and search coil recordings across healthy subjects and patients with a wide range of previously identified peripheral vestibular deficits (MacDougall et al. 2009).

They do not doubt the efficacy of the head impulse test (HIT) as a useful bedside test to identify peripheral vestibular deficits. But they believe that such a deficit of the vestibulo-ocular reflex (VOR) may not be diagnosed because corrective saccades cannot always be detected by simple observation. They believe that the scleral search coil technique should be the gold standard for HIT measurements. But one must remember that it is not practical for routine testing or in acute patients, because they are required to wear an uncomfortable contact lens.

In their study they recorded the horizontal HIT simultaneously with vHIT (250 Hz) and search coils (1,000 Hz) in 8 normal subjects, 6 patients with vestibular neuritis, 1 patient after unilateral intratympanic gentamicin and 1 patient with bilateral gentamicin vestibulotoxicity. Their results showed that simultaneous video and search coil recordings of eye movements were closely comparable (average concordance correlation coefficient $r(c) = 0.930$). Mean VOR gains measured with search coils and video were not significantly different in normal ($p = 0.107$) and patients ($p = 0.073$). With these groups, the sensitivity and specificity of both the reference and index test were 1.0 (95 % confidence interval 0.69–1.0). vHIT measures detected both overt and covert saccades as accurately as coils.

These research workers therefore concluded that video head impulse test is equivalent to search coils in identifying peripheral vestibular deficits but easier to use in clinics, even in patients with acute vestibular neuritis.

2.8   Fukuda and Unterberger's Test

This is one of the commonest and the simplest clinical test that we use in our daily practice, and find it to be a satisfactory indicator in giddy patients.

In this test, the patient is asked to walk straight with the closed eyes thus removing the ocular sensory element of the postural control. The patient with normal vestibular activity should walk straight without drifting away from the straight line, but in a case of peripheral vestibular disease, he drifts away towards the weaker vestibular organ.

2.9   Romberg's Test

It is a commonly performed test designed to check out the functioning of the proprioceptive impulses sending message about the movement of the distal peripheral locomotor elements, texture of the floor, any changes in the surface, etc. The information is transmitted through the posterior columns, to the cerebellum, while sharing the vital information about the peripheral environment to the vestibular system through the vestibulo-spinal pathways. Thus, this simple and extremely practical test can check out the functioning of the peripheral proprioceptive and exteroceptive reflexes, the cerebellum and the vestibular apparatus. The patient is asked to maintain balance with feet placed in a juxtaposition on a level footing with open eyes. If he fails to maintain the balance on removing the ocular input by closing the eyes, the test is declared positive for imbalance.

2.10   Past Pointing

It is a test that takes only a couple of minutes and is most routinely performed in an otolaryngology clinic. One common way of performing this test is to ask the patient to reach the index finger of the examiner with eyes closed with his right and left index finger alternating several times while the examiner holds his index finger in the middle and at comfortable distance. Theoretically it means that if the lesion is uncompensated and peripheral in nature, the ocular factor having been eliminated with the closure of eye, his perception of the distance and the object may be distorted. If the disease is unilateral, he tends to outshoot the target or simply drift away in the opposite direction, most likely to the healthy ear. This test has certain limitations and can only be used as an indicator towards a peripheral pathology, demanding further tests such as the calorimetric.

2.11   Dix–Hallpike Test

It is one of the original tests for vertigo that has stood the test of time. It is commonly employed in confirming a state of BPPV. The patient is requested to sit on an examining couch; after explaining the procedure his head is made to lie down in a supine position and head lowered to below the body level and rotated by 45° to one side. Nystagmus is to be checked in this position for 30–60 s as well as the patient asked about any subjective dizziness. If the patient feels dizzy and nystagmic beat is observed, the test is labelled to be positive. If repeated after brief interval, the nystagmus should not recur as against a central pathology, while each time the

Hallpike test is carried out, the nystagmus will reappear. Thus, the former is called a fatigue-able and the later non-fatigue-able nystagmus. Besides, in the BPPV the nystagmus will be directed towards the uppermost ear and ipsilateral in a central lesion such as a brainstem pathology. The procedure is repeated on the opposite ear after a brief resting period.

Dix–Hallpike test is one of the commonest clinical tests employed in the diagnosis of vertigo. It is also one of the oldest tests used by clinicians in differentiating between peripheral and central vertigo and has certainly stood the test of time.

The Dix–Hallpike manoeuvre involves the execution of the following basic steps. The patient is explained the manoeuvre and the head is rotated 45° to the right with eyes open while the patient is sitting on the examination couch. The physician holds the head and briskly takes the patient from a sitting to a supine posture so that the head is maintained hanging about 20° below the couch. This position is maintained for 30 s. The same exercise is then repeated on the opposite side. Throughout the manoeuvre the physician must continue to observe the eyes for nystagmus and ask the patient for subjective dizziness.

The peripheral nystagmus is indicative of a vestibular pathology. It has a latency period of about 3–30 s which is classically absent in central nystagmus. Another variable to be noted is the intensity of vertigo. It is quite severe in peripheral and relatively mild in central cases of vertigo.

Perhaps the most salient difference is in terms of duration of nystagmus initiated by the Dix–Hallpike manoeuvre. It is fatigue-able in peripheral vertigo and lasts about 50–55 s approximately and is non-fatigue-able in central causes lasting more than a minute. It means that on repeating the head manoeuvre, the peripheral nystagmus should not reappear, but a central nystagmus continues to reappear each time the manoeuvre is performed. Another important observations that peripheral nystagmus is contralateral in direction and central is ipsilateral in its direction.

Since the patients with central vertigo need further evaluation, it is essential that one must note for any telltale signs of central nervous system involvement, such as cranial nerve palsies.

The role of this useful clinical test was highlighted in a study conducted by Philips et al. (2009) involving 100 patients presenting with vertigo. It was found out that 60 patients had an abnormal vestibular assessment and 11 patients had BPPV as the sole diagnosis, but 9 of them did not have a Dix–Hallpike manoeuvre performed on them in the clinic. Furthermore, 76 % of those referred for vestibular rehabs had an abnormal electrophysiological assessment. They certainly hit the nail on its head, when they recommended that the patients must have a Dix–Hallpike manoeuvre performed prior to referral to the vestibular lab. We perform this simple and least time-consuming test routinely as is indeed do most physicians dealing with vertigo. It is simply invaluable in confirming a possible vestibular lesion, in a few minutes, and can save unnecessary and expensive investigations. We feel that it should be part of a routine evaluation in almost all patients except for any physical contraindications like cervical osteoarthritis or obvious CVS disease.

King and colleagues (2006) designed an automated mental alerting task that could be utilised when performing vestibular testing on a broad range of populations, including difficult cases like hard of hearing patients. They developed a device that utilised the vibrotactile stimuli output to two vibrators placed on the subjects' left leg and responded to activation of two momentary pushbuttons controlled by them. This was followed by the instruction to the subjects to carry out three mental alerting conditions, defined as no task, verbal task or vibrotactile task. They further describe the details of the procedure inferring that the vibrotactile tasking device (VTD) is an effective alternative means of providing mental alerting during vestibular testing, especially that of calorimetry. We have no practical experience of this application and wait to learn more about it in due course of time.

Hoffman et al. (1999) conducted a structured literature synthesis on the aetiology, prognosis and diagnostic evaluation of dizziness, with a view to suggest a primary care approach to evaluating this symptom. Several studies were identified from Medline searches (1966–1996) and a manual search of bibliographies from retrieved articles. The most common aetiologies for dizziness were found to be peripheral vestibulopathies (35–55 % of patients) and psychiatric disorders (10–25 % of patients). Cerebrovascular disease (5 %) and brain tumours (<1 %) were infrequent. The significance of history taking and a thorough clinical examination was duly supplemented by this study, as it led to a diagnosis in about 75 % of patients. At least 10 % of patients eluded diagnosis.

It was also noted that in most situations, the symptoms were self-limited without an increased risk of mortality.

The research concluded that dizziness is usually a benign, self-limiting complaint. When a diagnosis can be made, a careful history and physical examination will usually identify the probable cause. Cardiovascular, neurological and laboratory testing should be guided by the clinical evaluation. In the author's opinion rigorous studies are needed to determine the accuracy and utility of specialised vestibular testing. We concur with this study and once again bring our point home that a comprehensive history and a thorough clinical examination are the fundamental factors in the diagnosis of vertigo. To say that the diagnosis of vertigo is a cerebral exercise may not be untrue.

Cohen and Kimball (2008) looked at the efficacy *and* reliability of current tests for identifying individuals with vestibular vertigo. They compared the scores of normal cohorts and patients on the Berg Balance Scale (Berg), Dynamic Gait Index (DGI), Timed Up and Go (TUG), Computerised Dynamic Posturography Sensory Organisation Test (SOT) and a new obstacle avoidance test called the Functional Mobility Test (FMT).

The study was performed in an outpatient vestibular laboratory at a tertiary care centre. The main outcome measures were the sensitivity of tests to patients and specificity to normal cohorts. It was noted that after they were adjusted for age, the Berg, TUG, DGI and FMT had moderate sensitivity and specificity. It was also observed that Sensory Organisation Test had moderately high sensitivity and specificity and SOT and FMT, when combined together, had high sensitivity and moderate specificity.

Therefore, tests like standing and walking in a balance clinic, used for assessing the chances of falling are not as efficient for screening of vestibular disorders as SOT. These research workers believe that SOT combined with FMT is a better test for arriving at a diagnosis. These two tests are simple and can be employed in a balance clinic. We do not have any personal experience of these tests, but would certainly like to try them out in our clinical practice, as we are ably supported by a fine vestibular lab.

The writers believe that when screening the patients for vestibular disorders, particularly if objective diagnostic tests of the vestibular system are not feasible, the tests of both standing and walking balance may give the most information about community-dwelling patients.

These tests may also indicate the presence of subclinical problems of balance in community-dwelling, asymptomatic adults. This particular application could be of much value in a community practice.

It is a common observation that people with balance disorders have difficulty with transitional movements, such as the sit-to-stand movement. A valid and feasible tool is needed to help clinicians quantify the ability of such people to perform transitional movements. Therefore, Whitney et al. (2005) conducted a research with the purpose of describing the concurrent and discriminative validity of data obtained with the Five-Times-Sit-to-Stand Test (FTSST), against the Activities-specific Balance Confidence Scale (ABC) and the Dynamic Gait Index (DGI). These variables are basically research orientated and we as clinicians look towards our scientist colleagues for interpretation of the results in studies employing them. Our main job is to apply the knowledge thus gained in our patients to serve them with the latest knowledge duly complimented with matching skills. It is essential for a clinician to keep refreshed and updated in all matters that concern him. This study is valid, specific and useful; hence, it is included here.

The investigators in this study compared 81 normal subjects and 93 dizzy patients. Each subject was asked to stand from a chair five times as quickly as possible. The ABC and DGI scores were recorded. The results of their study showed that the dizzy subjects performed the FTSST more slowly than controls. Discriminant analysis demonstrated that the FTSST correctly identified 65 % vertiginous subjects, the ABC identified 80 % and the DGI identified 78 %. It was observed that ability of the FTSST to identify dizzy subjects was better for relatively younger subjects, i.e. 60 years of age.

The conclusion was that the FTSST displayed properties with discriminative and concurrent validity that made this test potentially useful in making a clinical decision. One must, however, add that overall the tests, namely, ABC and the DGI are better than the FTSST at discriminating between subjects with and without vertigo.

In a busy ENT clinic, it is not possible to perform many of these tests; however, a clinician must know the latest research in the field to apply the most appropriate test in his practice.

2.12 Oscillopsia

It is more commonly seen by the ophthalmologists and neuro-physicians than by us in the ENT clinics. This clinical entity is best described by the patient presenting with blurred vision as an 'image that seems to move' (Blender 1965). It may be a peculiar movement which the patient may describe as bobbing, dancing, jumping, etc. In other words, the patient feels that the object in focus does not seem to stand still. In clinical practice, we have seen a few cases of oscillopsia, with vague description of images floating or running away etc. Most are usually referred to the ophthalmologists and neurologists for further investigation and management. Sometimes, however, the picture may be confusing if the presenting features are those of vertigo, dizziness or similar symptoms. Obviously nystagmus would be seen in these patients, but it certainly merits vestibular investigations to rule out a peripheral or central vestibular pathology.

2.13   Nijmegen Scoring

It is a chart comprising of numerous questions employed to differentiate between genuine vertigo caused by peripheral vestibular disease and a false sense of imbalance caused by hyperventilation or a panic attack. A list of observations are made by the vestibular scientist to rule out hyperventilation as a possible cause of dizziness. It is a well-documented fact that through hyperventilation, one may wash out the CO_2 from one's blood. It may reduce, even critically drop, the $PaCO_2$ levels. CO_2 is the basic stimulant for respiration to function normally. Washing out the CO_2 leads to shallow breathing, resulting in fall in oxygen saturation (PaO_2), sometimes resulting in hypoxia of the brain. In turn, it may result in a feeling of dizziness, even a momentary loss of consciousness. Hyperventilation could be brought about by psychological rather vestibular reasons. Anxiety leading to hyperventilation resulting in panic attacks may be caused by certain pulmonary and cardiac ailments also.

Abnormal somatic sensations are felt by these patients which further aggravate the panic state. Some of these patients may actually feel quite unsteady on their feet. Some might even show rolling of the eyes and an obvious picture of anxiety and stress. We use the questionnaire included here. A score of 23 out of 64 suggests an affirmative diagnosis of hyperventilation syndrome. It is a differential diagnosis of dizziness in some cases. Those positive may require relaxation exercises, often with quite encouraging outcomes.

2.13.1 Nijmegen Questionnaire

Scoring:
Never = 0
Rarely = 1
Sometimes = 2
Often = 3
Very often = 4
Chest pain
Feeling tense
Blurred vision

Dizzy spells
Confusion
Faster breathing
Shortness of breath
Tightness across the chest
Bloated stomach
Tingling sensations in fingers
Difficulty in deep berating
Stiff fingers
Tightness around the mouth
Cold, clammy hands or feet
Palpitations
Anxiety

Computers have become inseparable component of our daily lives. In medicine as in many other fields of science, this tool has all but revolutionised the whole philosophy of research. The application of computers in the field of otolaryngology has been almost three decades old. It was employed in a research recently as described here. Computer-aided vestibular autorotational testing of the vestibulo-ocular reflex in senile vestibular dysfunction was the subject of a study conducted a few months ago (Chiu et al. 2010).

In this study, the authors confirmed that studies have already investigated vestibulo-ocular reflex (VOR) responses in elderly subjects, mostly at low frequencies (<1 Hz) during passive head turns or continuous active head turns in a rotational chair. However, natural head movements usually occur at frequencies above 1 Hz and at varying rates, rather than at continuously increasing rates as tested in most studies to date.

The aim of this study was to compare VOR responses within or between normal and bilateral peripheral vestibular hypofunction (BPVH) in elderly subjects with a computer-based programme incorporating random active high-frequency head movements.

It was found out that the VAT paradigm can be improved by using concurrent horizontal and vertical moving targets. The VOR phase may be useful for differentiating VAT responses between BPVH and healthy elderly subjects. Moreover, the results of this study demonstrate that gains in VOR at different frequencies of head shaking and asymmetry during different test conditions can be useful parameters for within-group assessment.

2.14 Cerebellar Tests

If one suspects a cerebellar disorder, then tests for dysdiadokinesia, dysarthria and ataxia should be carried out as described in many books of clinical neurology. It is beyond the scope of this book to discuss all those clinical and laboratory evaluations. Some of the fundamental tests we routinely perform in our patients for evaluation of gait and CNS are mentioned earlier in this book. As a matter of fact, in our practice, we involve our neurology colleagues in the diagnosis and management of our dizzy patients quite regularly. It goes without saying that we as ENT specialists have a secondary role in the diagnosis and treatment of cerebellar vertigo. We are, however, always ready to help our colleagues out in excluding or confirming an audio-vestibular pathology. All clinicians know that despite the compartmentalisation of medicine, due to specialisation, a holistic approach and team effort always yields better results. It should not be a matter of ego to request a colleague when needed without unduly overburdening them either. An ethical practice must remain the motto of every clinician, and the fundamental principles of beneficence compounded with non-maleficence must remain in the forefront.

2.15   Haematological Tests

Usually it is the general practitioner who would carry out the routine blood tests before referral for an otolaryngological opinion. Sometimes these tests may not have been requested and the clinical otolaryngologist may thus be obliged to do so.

Full blood picture is essential to establish the baseline and exclude common causes of light-headedness such as anaemia, a blood glucose test and a urinalysis are absolutely essential to exclude an underlying metabolic condition such as diabetes a common cause of fainting attack, light-headedness even loss of consciousness. Of course in such situations the patient would require referral to the physicians for further management.

Hypercholesterolaemia and hyperlipidaemia are also common conditions seen in many patients. One may request a lipid profile as it could be a possible contributor towards light-headedness and dizziness. Most such patients are either already diagnosed or will be diagnosed in due course of time, as they may require long-term physical care. Vitamin D and B12 deficiencies are common in the Asian diaspora and thalassaemia minor is a fairly known finding in the Afro-Caribbean population. The role of an otolaryngologist in such situations is only secondary. Nevertheless, in an ageing population in Britain, many such patients are referred to an ENT clinic for excluding a vestibular cause of vertiginous symptoms. Often enough in such patients, an MRI may show ischaemic changes of mild or minor nature in the basal ganglia or the cerebral cortex. Not too similarly, demyelinising conditions may indeed be diagnosed on radiological investigation.

Diagnostic tests are adventitious and can only supplement the physician in reaching a diagnosis. The pivotal role of a clinician in the diagnosis of vertiginous patients is further highlighted by Polensek et al. (2008) who found out that vestibular impairment was an underlying cause in as many as 45 % of people complaining of dizziness. In this study, computerised medical records of all patients receiving an ICD-9 diagnosis code for dizziness, including benign paroxysmal positional vertigo, Meniere's disease and reduced vestibular function over a 6-month period, was reviewed.

It was a fairly large study, involving 157 patients selected from a total sample of over 400 cohorts. About two-thirds of providers (69 %) used the patient's description of the dizziness for identifying the cause; however, significant variability was evident across disciplines, ranging from 84 % of audiologists asking for a description of the dizziness to only 33 % of geriatricians asking. A vast proportion (89 %) of providers did not evaluate a patient for BPPV by examining for positional nystagmus. Dix–Hallpike is such a simple and quick test, which can save many a missed diagnosis. At least in our practice, we employ it nearly all the time. What was more interesting about this study was that the primary care physicians referred 22 % of dizzy patients to a neurologist; the geriatricians referred 17 %, and emergency physicians referred only 16 %. The patients were not routinely screened for vestibular impairment, which as we know is a main contributor to the menace of dizziness. This study duly highlights the validity of argument that each case of vertigo is a clinical entity in its own right and demands a comprehensive history taking and a thorough clinical examination, keeping in mind that peripheral vestibular causes are indeed the commonest cause of dizziness in a clinical setting.

It was concluded in the study that based on available recommended practices, many factors may be contributing to the underdiagnosis and early treatment. We feel one of them is an improper clinical workup.

Their results highlighted a need for effective dissemination of guidelines to improve health-care quality, increase awareness of medical risks and enhance patient access to appropriate treatment.

Therefore, the role of a family physician in acquiring and disseminating such knowledge as indeed of the ENT departments through relevant pamphlets, fliers, CME programmes, seminars and other educational or informative tools is simply indispensable.

2.15.1 Other Lab Investigations

Routine urinalysis is carried out in our clinics, as it rules out many clinical reasons for dizziness, such as diabetes. Usually the patients referred to us have their clinical day available to us on the Clinical Data Archives (CDA) on our computers, and we certainly use them on a regular basis. In some places, if such a facility is not available, family physician would normally have carried out the essential lab workup, before referring a patient for an ENT consultation. Every clinician knows the importance of the very basic lab investigations that can help exclude many and confirm the relevant findings, which are duly flagged up on the CDA.

2.16 Radiology

Radiology is an inseparable component of a clinician's diagnostic arsenal. In otology it has played the most significant role since the early days when brain abscess was a common complication of acute fulminating or chronic suppurative otitis media. Later on the evolution of radiology brought in an era of tomography and polytomograms. Some fine radiologists in the early 1970s could pick up the minutest of pathologies such as the dehiscence of the tegmen tympani or a labyrinthine fistula on these tomograms. There were some pundits who could actually delineate the course of the facial nerve all along the middle ear and parts of the petrous bones showing any congenital or acquired dehiscence of the facial bony capsule.

The CT scans have all but revolutionised the diagnosis of the chronic ear disease. The faintest of pathologies that may escape a clinician's sight will be picked up by the radiologist. Cholesteatomas and their impending disasters are routinely diagnosed with the CT scans as indeed other pathologies involving the temporal bones. However, a word of warning may be mentioned here that the radiology must be complimented with the clinical evaluation of a patient, as sometimes a scan may show a cholesteatoma in the attic region, but clinically there may be no sign of an active ear disease. In such situations it is best advised to observe the patient and review the situation on timely basis. Silent cholesteatomas are not unknown and there are some cases where the ear disease may have burnt itself out leaving the marks on the scans but no activity per se.

In congenital anomalies of the ear, such as agenesis, atresia, partial atresia, malformation of the middle ear ossicles, and cochlear agenesis, malformation or distorted formation, i.e. anomalies which may be part of a syndrome, nothing can beat the CT scanning.

CT scans have some limitations, which are fairly compensated by the magnetic resonance imaging. The latter also has a few limitations such as it cannot be employed in those patients who may carry a metallic prosthesis in their body or a cardiac pacemaker. Therefore, the clinician may decide which radiological investigation would suit the patient best. Generally speaking CT is good for bony disease like suspected erosion of the temporal bone or the ossicles, and the MRI is ideal for checking out the soft tissue pathology. One major reason for worries in the diagnosis of vertigo is the uncommon but sinister condition of an acoustic neuroma.

As far as its diagnosis is concerned, undoubtedly imaging has changed the complexion of the game altogether. We have discussed the application of imaging in our cases as and when required. Magnetic resonance imaging has not only eliminated the factor of doubt and missing out a pathology but also immensely helped in picking up these tumours at very early stages. And that by itself is no mean feat. There were times in not too distant past that the conventional X-ray was requested for highlighting the anatomical status of the internal auditory meatus in a suspected case of an acoustic neuroma one looked for the slightest telltale sign of expansion or distortion of the IAM. If found it was described as 'funnelling' and an almost certain sign of an intracanalicular tumour having breached the confines of the internal meatus only to invade the cerebellopontine angle. Of course in more advanced tumours, the diagnosis was mainly clinical like the presence of facial nerve paralysis as well as the vestibulocochlear involvement. Polytomography was another tool often used in many centres; one dreads to think though as to how many early tumours may have been missed out. Thanks to the MRI, duly supplemented with a gadolinium contrast medium study, our colleagues in the department of radiology have picked up the tiniest of tumours and have indeed excelled in their art of sleuthing these nasty albeit slow-growing tumours.

Korres et al. (2009) looked at the diagnostic role of ENG and MRI in a population in which the history and clinical examination had failed to provide a conclusive diagnosis of the origin, i.e. peripheral or central. It was a retrospective study on 102 patients. Following a detailed history, an ENT as well as neurotological assessment was carried out. It was followed by a PTA, an ABR, an ENG and an MRI. It was a fairly comprehensive study which showed that the ENG contributed to the confirmation of a diagnosis in 52 %, whereas MRI did the same in a significantly less proportion of cases.

Korres points out that many clinicians underestimate the importance of an ENG in establishing the cause of vertigo. MRI no doubt is invaluable in the diagnosis of a central cause of vertigo, but in this study it failed to contribute to the etiological diagnosis of 98/102 patients in a population prone to developing central vestibular disorders. And that is a major factor to note. Korres also mentioned that the ENG on the other hand contributed to reaching a diagnosis in 53/102 patients. This author, therefore, concluded that electronystagmography was the most useful tool in the diagnosis of vestibular vertigo.

Despite that, we believe an MRI is an indispensable tool amongst the diagnostic aids required in many cases of vertigo, particularly of suspicious nature.

2.17 Vestibular Investigations

Carefully taken history still remains the cornerstone of a physician's arsenal. Detailed vestibular investigations are however sometimes indicated in those cases where the diagnosis is either difficult or unsatisfactory. Most cases of imbalance settle down without even referral to a specialist clinic. Those that need further evaluation are certainly the cases that have either failed to resolve or are posing some difficulty in management.

A clinician is well poised to perform clinical assessment for disequilibrium; however, more detailed investigations are required in some situations. The vestibular lab is better equipped with the logistics and trained personnel to do such tests. Komazec looked at the clinician's role in the management of dizziness (Lemajic-Komazec and Komazec 2006).

They remind us that maintenance of balance depends upon receiving afferent sensory information from several sensory systems: vestibular, optical and proprioceptive. Bioelectric signals, generated by body movements in the semicircular canals and in otolithic apparatus are transmitted via the vestibular nerve to the vestibular nucleus. All four vestibular nuclei, located bilaterally in medial longitudinal fasciculus, are linked with central nervous system structures. These central nervous system structures are involved in maintaining visual stability, spatial orientation and balance control. Nystagmus is a result of afferent signal balance disorders.

Nystagmus due to peripheral lesions is a conjugate nystagmus, because there is a bilateral central connection. Lesions above the vestibular nuclei induce deficits in synchronisation and conjugation of eye movements; thus, the nystagmus is dissociated.

They concur with the universally accepted observation that in peripheral vestibular disorders spontaneous nystagmus is rhythmic, associated, horizontal-rotatory or horizontal, with subjective sensation of dizziness which decreases with time and harmonic signs whose direction coincides with the slow phase of nystagmus, and it is associated with mild disorders during pendular stimulation with statistically significant vestibular hypofunction.

Spontaneous nystagmus in central vestibular lesions is severe, dissociated, rotatory or vertical, without changes related to optical suppression; if vestibular symptoms are present, they are nonharmonic.

In central disorders, findings after thermal stimulation are either normal or pathological, with dysrhythmias and inhibition in pendular stimulation. Calorimetry is the cornerstone of vestibular evaluation, but it may not be required in all the cases, according to these workers.

The introduction of Videonystagmography (VNG) and vestibular-evoked myogenic potentials (VEMP) have changed the picture of diagnostic evaluation to a great extent.

VEMP is just beginning to gain grounds and promises to be an indispensable tool in the future. Electronystagmography was very popular until recently, but is now being superseded by the VNG. In ENG the vertical and horizontal eye movements are recorded indirectly through the use of corneo-retinal potential via the electrodes placed at each lateral canthus with the common electrode planted on the forehead. A few illustrations are included in this clinical guide.

The VNG is more appropriate and precise as the eye movements are picked up directly through the infrared video cameras. Besides, compared with the ENG, the tracing is neater and more specific, recording the most delicate of nystagmic beat not easily discernible by an observer's eye. Many fine beats cannot be picked up by magnifying aids like the Frenzel's glasses. Besides, electronic equipment gives precise results and a clinician must employ them for a precise diagnosis, when required.

The purpose of VNG just like the ENG is to identify the focal point of pathology in the vestibular end organs. Therefore, certain specific tests are performed to reach that goal. They include tests for both horizontal and vertical gaze, assessment of saccades, recording of head shaking movements leading to ocular movement, positional testing and if indicated calorimetry. Details of all these tests are available in standard textbooks.

Some of the vestibular tests performed in our lab are described in the relevant case reports. Suffice it to say that from the early day of Cawthorne, Citron, Dix and Hallpike, vestibulometry has come a long way. The main focus these days is to employ only the highly sophisticated, state-of-the-art electronic equipments such as the VNG, VEMP and vHIT to literally pinpoint a lesion in the tiniest corner of the vestibular apparatus.

2.17.1   VNG in the Investigation of Vertigo (Figs. 2.1, 2.2, 2.3, 2.4 and 2.5)

We use it in our vestibular labs on a routine basis. We have an excellent team of scientists, who help us in the interpretation of the results. We have ample reasons to believe that along with the clinical evaluation, the VNG makes definitive diagnosis easier.

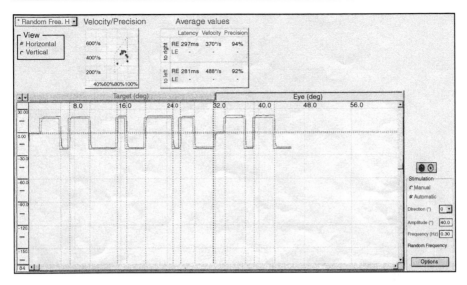

Fig. 2.1 VNG recording of random frequency horizontal saccades in a normal subject. Eye movements recorded with video goggles while the subject watches a moving target projected onto a screen in front of him. The *y* axis illustrates the degree of deviation from central gaze along a horizontal line. Zero degrees is the straight-ahead position. Movement to the right is shown as positive, i.e. upwards on the scale, and movement to the left as negative. The *x* axis represents time in seconds. The *green trace* shows the movement of the target and the *red trace* shows the eye movement of the subject. The tester examines the general morphology of the trace for abnormalities and specifically the values of latency, velocity and accuracy. These are determined by the software and the velocity and accuracy of each saccade is plotted on a summary graph above the trace. The *dotted diamond* area on this graph illustrates the normal range defined by the software

Videonystagmography (VNG) is a very specialised field and the reader is best advised to consult standard textbooks on vestibular investigations for further details. In brief, this technology enables us to record the eye movements which are involved in the maintenance of proper eye function. They are the smooth pursuits which outline the ability to stabilise a visual gaze in pursuit of a moving object and the saccades. The recordings of saccades enable us to judge and evaluate the capability of the eye to jump from one object to another effectively, accurately and efficiently. Saccades are employed by the oculo-visual system to perceive and interpret images smoothly.

Recordings of some salient and common conditions seen in our vestibular lab are described here.

2.17.2 VEMP

The vestibular-evoked myogenic potential (VEMP) is a relatively new test, which is being investigated at present in patients with specific vestibular disorders. It is a biphasic response elicited by loud clicks or tone bursts recorded from the tonically con-

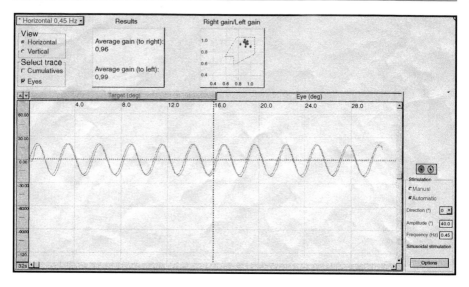

Fig. 2.2 Videonystagmography recording of horizontal smooth pursuit in a normal subject. Eye movements are recorded with video goggles while the subject watches a projected target swing from side to side horizontally onto a screen in front of them. The *y* axis illustrates the degrees of deviation from central gaze along a horizontal line. Zero degrees is the straight-ahead position. Movement to the right is shown as positive, i.e. upwards on the scale, and movement to the left as negative. The *x* axis represents time in seconds. The *green trace* shows the movement of the target and the *red trace* shows the eye movement of the subject. A normal subject should be able to follow the target smoothly to both sides without the use of saccadic movements. The gain of the subject's eye movements is also measured and plotted in the figure above the recording trace. The normal range for gain defined by the software is illustrated by the *dotted arrowhead* area

tracted sternomastoid muscle, which is the only source available to assess the function of saccule and the lower part of vestibular nerve (Cal and Bahmad 2009). Rauch in his review article claims that VEMP is the only clinically feasible way to measure function of the saccule. Interest in this diagnostic tool is rapidly gaining significance particularly in the evaluation of third window disorders and for monitoring Meniere's disease. Rauch believes that much has still to be done in this exciting field, but the field of VEMP continues to evolve and soon it should be a routine test (Rauch 2006).

Sakakura et al. (2005) described a new and innovative method of recording a VEMP. They acknowledged that vestibular-evoked myogenic potential (VEMP) has been used to test the vestibulo-collic reflex. However, they argued that VEMP is not stable in elderly patients because of their weak musculature. Therefore, they recorded VEMP on median neck extensor muscles with weak muscular contraction. Thirty-one normal subjects and 56 patients with vertigo or hearing loss were tested in a seated or prone position without muscular tension. Different electrodes were placed on the median surface at the palpable bottom of the occipital bone. Their study showed a clear negative peak at 13 ms on normal subjects, with reversed polarity compared with VEMP on the sternocleidomastoid muscle. This potential is defined as VEMP caused by the proper latencies, dependency of the strength on sound stimulation and independence of hearing ability. In the cases of acoustic neuroma, onset latencies were prolonged or nonexistent. The responses on neck exten-

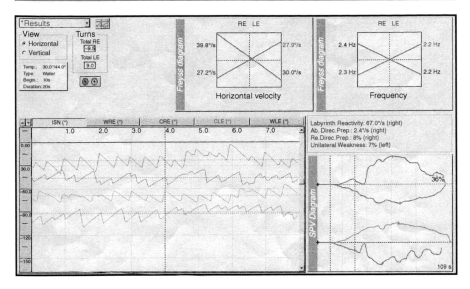

Fig. 2.3 Bithermal water caloric results recorded using videonystagmography for a subject with normal vestibular function. Image illustrates the nystagmus of peak slow phase velocity of horizontal nystagmus provoked by each irrigation (warm right ear = *red*, warm left ear = *pink*, cool right ear = *blue*, cool left ear = *green*). The Freyss diagram of horizontal velocity shows the numerical values of the peak slow phase velocity for each irrigation, allowing calculation of canal paresis and direction preponderance. The nystagmus provoked in this case is robust and approximately equal bilaterally

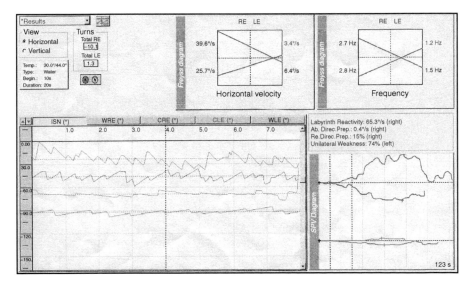

Fig. 2.4 Bithermal water caloric results recorded using videonystagmography for a subject with a left-side peripheral vestibular weakness. This subject was later diagnosed with Meniere's disease. Image illustrates the nystagmus of peak slow phase velocity of horizontal nystagmus provoked by each irrigation (warm right ear = *red*, warm left ear = *pink*, cool right ear = *blue*, cool left ear = *green*). The Freyss diagram of horizontal velocity shows the numerical values of the peak slow phase velocity for each irrigation, allowing calculation of canal paresis and direction preponderance. In this case it can be seen that the irrigations on the left ear provoked a significantly lower peak slow phase velocity

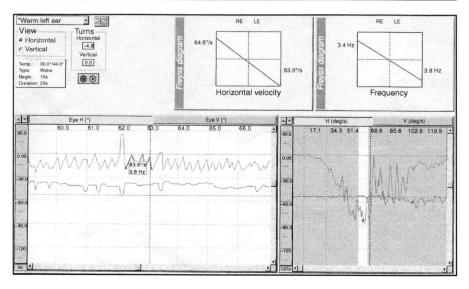

Fig. 2.5 Warm water caloric videonystagmography result for a subject with possible vestibular hyperfunction. The figure shows where the peak of the nystagmus has been measured and a peak slow phase velocity of over 80°/s was recorded. The Freyss diagram of horizontal velocity above the recording shows that both the right and left warm irrigations produced elevated responses. The diagnosis of vestibular hyperfunction can be controversial and completion of the cool irrigations in addition to the warm may be necessary to make this diagnosis; however, this subject withdrew consent before the test was completed. An MRI of the head is mandatory in such a patient

sor muscles could not be recorded on some elderly patients. They believe that this new method of recording VEMP is less invasive and suitable for elderly patients.

No doubt the world will look into this yet another addition to the arsenal of a clinician with much interest, as the burden of disease and disability caused by ageing population continues to grow.

Increasingly a large number of research scientists are exploring finer ways of localising the site of pathology in the vestibular organ. It is exciting to note that we are now entering into the hitherto unapproachable territories. Not just the techniques but the application of modern as well as time-honoured subjects like physics, arithmetic and trigonometry by our research colleagues is opening new avenues every day. It is obviously up to a clinician to harness them to benefit his patients.

Viatl et al. carried out a study designed to evaluate a novel test for dynamic visual acuity (DVA) that employs algorithm for changing the size of Landolt rings presented during active or passive head impulses and to compare the results with search-coil head impulse testing. It was a prospective study that concluded that dynamic visual acuity testing with Landolt rings that are adaptively changed in size enables detection of peripheral vestibular dysfunction in a fast and simpler way (Vital et al. 2010).

Donnellan et al. (2010) studied the frequency tuning of bone-conducted soundevoked myogenic potentials recording them from the extraocular muscles. It was a small sample of only nine cohorts. The acoustic tone bursts (57 dB nHL, 8 ms plateau, 1 ms rise/fall alternating polarity) with frequencies from 250 to 2,000 Hz were delivered by the oscillator placed on the left mastoid process. They were instructed to sit upright looking straight at a fixed point, in a gaze. Then these workers recorded BOVEMP from surface electrodes placed at four locations around the right eye, namely, superior, inferior, medial and lateral regions, and referenced to an electrode placed at the level of seventh cervical vertebra. They then amplified the signals (1,000 gain) from the electrodes and sampled at 10 kHz averaged over 500 repetitions.

Their study resulted in demonstrating the presence of short latency biphasic potentials at each of the four recording sites around the eye. Specific technical details are given by the authors, which are rather difficult for us clinicians to comprehend, but are mentioned here to give a fuller picture to the reader. They found out that the average latency of the first peak (negative) and the sound peak (positive) was 15.7 ± 0.3 ms and 23.3 ± 0.5 ms, respectively. They observed a few other variables and concluded that since the frequency using for the bone-anchored sound-evoked OVEMP (BOVEMP) was different from that of the air-conducted sound-evoked OVEMP (AOVEMP), they hypothesised that the BOVEMP and AOVEMP are generated by activation of different vestibular end organs.

Many cases of viral vestibular vertigo may present in combination with hearing loss. Theoretically it is understood that after an acute phase is over, if the hearing returns to normal, it would be labelled as vestibulitis or more appropriately vestibular neuritis. It basically implies that only the vestibular part of the vestibulocochlear nerve is affected. On the other hand, if the hearing loss persists, it would be labelled as a case of labyrinthitis, meaning thereby that only the cochlear component of the eighth cranial nerve was involved.

Some cases of sudden hearing loss may have no associated symptoms like tinnitus or vertigo at all. And since no definite aetiology can be established, they are often labelled as 'idiopathic' sudden hearing loss or deafness. Any loss which is total is called deafness, but a loss less than total would be mild (20–40 dB), moderate (40–70 dB), severe (70–90 dB) or profound (above 90 dB), depending upon the intensity of hearing loss in decibels. The speech range tested on PTA is between 250 and 4,000 Hz, and the acceptable levels for normal hearing threshold is between 0 and 20 dB(A).

Korres et al. (2009) investigated the diagnostic role of VEMP in assessment of vestibular function in cases of sudden idiopathic hearing loss. They found it to be an exceptionally useful addition to the arsenal of diagnostic tests. This technical advancement in vestibular investigations is very exciting, but still quite new and may take some time before it is freely available in most if not all vestibular labs.

2.18   Video Head Impulse Test (vHIT)

This is the latest entry in the field of vestibular investigations. It is a rotational test designed to measure the eye movement responses to small, brief, passive, unpredictable, natural acceleration head turns to either side performed manually by the physician or the vestibular scientist while the patient is instructed to fix the gaze on an earth-fixed dot on the front wall in the vestibular lab. The fixed dot is placed about 1 m from the patient in front of his eyes.

In order to check out the function of the horizontal semicircular canals, approximately 20 horizontal head impulses are delivered manually. The details of the test and its methodology are beautifully described by Curthoys in this research paper. It is highly recommended to be read.

Curthoys also believes that vHIT may actually replace the traditional calorimetry in due course of time. He claims that calorimetry has many inherent problems. Some of which are well known to all clinicians such as contraindications due to infection, hypertension, presyncope, etc. The author has mentioned some unusual problems with calorimetry such as poor caloric responses despite normal semicircular canals due to anthropomorphic reasons etc.

This paper also describes a few limitations of this test, such as neck stiffness or inability to relax the neck muscles on request etc. Many of our case reports will display the same observation, as our vestibular colleagues either deferred (until the hypertension settled down) or cancelled a calorimetry (due to a stiff neck or osteoarthritis). One hopes that if an alternate procedure such as that described by Curthoys proves to be useful with satisfactory sensitivity and specificity, it will be duly appreciated. It is claimed to be extremely precise, efficient and least time-consuming. We know that the conventional calorimetry is neither absolutely precise to identify the lesion nor indeed economical both in terms of manpower and the lab time consumed. At present we find somewhat handicapped if the calorimetry is abandoned and clinical judgement alone has to guide us. In the current environment of evidence-based medicine, presence of an evidence makes a huge difference.

Obviously all those interested in managing the vertiginous patients would watch with interest further development of this test in the future.

2.19   Audiometry

Pure tone audiometry, tympanometry and various other audiological investigations are inseparable components of the diagnostic tools for vertigo. Most patients presenting with vertigo in an ENT clinic also have such symptoms as hearing impairment, tinnitus, otorrhoea, earache, blockage of the ear, muffled hearing or fluctuation of hearing.

The importance of history in the clinical diagnosis has been discussed earlier. One has to pay due attention to the intensity and variability of these symptoms. Of course each patient presenting with vertigo requires a battery of audiological tests. The Pure Tone Audiometry (PTA) is the very basic test that sets the fundamental standard of hearing level (Fig. 2.6).

If the PTA is normal, it goes in favour of excluding any significant otological cause of vertigo, but not entirely. For instance, a patient of vestibular neuritis may have normal PTA, but will have dizziness as well as nystagmus. However, if the patient has unilateral sensorineural loss with vertigo, especially with ipsilateral tinnitus, then an acoustic neuroma must be excluded with the help of an MRI of internal meati and cerebellopontine angle.

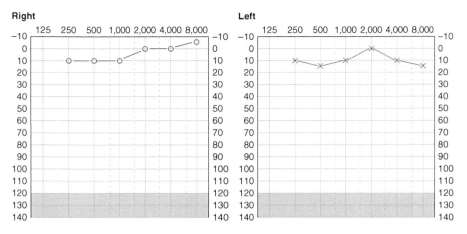

Fig. 2.6 Figure shows a normal pure tone audiogram (PTA). By convention the *red colour* code represents the hearing levels in the right and blue in the left ear. By the same convention an *o* represents air conduction in the right and an *x* in the left ear. The hearing levels in this audiogram show the hearing to stand between 10 and 20 dB(A) in the speech range (250–4,000 Hz)

In a case of bilateral sensorineural hearing loss, vertigo may be an important symptom, but non-otological causes such as cervicogenic vertigo or migrainous vertigo may come to mind as a differential diagnosis. If the patient is elderly, then presbyacusis with tinnitus and aches and pains in the neck may give an inclination of a non-ontological cause, requiring further evaluation. If the patient has normal PTA and vertigo is associated with either migraine or cluster headaches, specially a young female, one may ask if the symptoms are associated with the menstruation cycle, as premenstrual tension may present with migraine like headaches, dizziness and a normal PTA.

A patient presenting with acute vertigo, fluctuating hearing loss and tinnitus should be investigated as a case of Ménière's disease. The PTA in such a patient would show unilateral or bilateral sensorineural hearing loss. Its intensity may vary with the duration and longevity of Meniere's. During an attack, PTA would be below normal level in the affected ear. If the PTA is recorded during an intermission, the PTA would be normal or near normal, as Meniere's is known to leave the patient with some degree of residual sensorineural hearing loss, which tends to worsen progressively as the attacks keep relapsing.

If the patient had developed an acute volatile intense vertigo leading to total incapacitation during the attack which may last several weeks, the possibility is that the PTA remains unaffected on the ipsilateral side. When the patient had tinnitus and hearing impairment during the attack, it may show profound hearing loss (more than 90 dB) or total loss, i.e. deafness. Such a patient should have periodical audiological assessment. If the PTA shows gradual improvement in hearing with the passage of time, the diagnosis would be vestibular neuronitis alone or one with mild to moderate degree of cochlear involvement. If the PTA on successive recordings over several months shows no improvement, the cause of vertigo would be labelled as viral labyrinthitis, i.e. with the involvement of the cochlear component of the vestibulocochlear nerve.

Impedance audiometry is equally important in evaluation of a vertiginous patient. Its role is mainly directed towards the diagnosis of a problem in the middle ear or the Eustachian tube. It also checks out the movement of eardrum and the middle ear ossicles, in response to the pressure changes created in the external auditory canal. It also informs us about the pressure changes in the external auditory canal.

Glue ear or serous effusion in the middle ear is a common condition, particularly in children. It is a known cause of dizziness in that age group. In adults a patient presenting with Eustachian malfunction and dizziness will obviously show diminished middle ear pressure and some variation in compliance. Type A tympanogram shows normal middle ear pressure, normal mobility of the eardrum and the ossicles. Type B tympanogram may indicate a scarred eardrum, fluid in the middle ear or a perforated eardrum. Type A tympanogram rules out a middle ear cause such as Eustachian malfunction or effusion. Type C or a flat graph would be a strong indicator of middle ear pathology, otitis media with effusion alias a glue ear. In a case of ossicular discontinuity following a trauma, the PTA may show variable degrees of sensorineural loss, with typical changes in an impedance audiogram, such as high peak or total separation of the graph, i.e. inability of the two limbs to join at the peak.

Since paediatric vertigo is a more complex diagnostic issue than adults, we have preferred to briefly describe various audiological tests that are performed in our labs in the young population. Some children presenting with dizziness may require some of these tests.

In children presenting with vertigo, sometimes an ABR may be required to establish the cochlear function, though in infants a Visual Reinforcement Audiometry (VRA) and behavioural audiometry, distraction audiometry, etc. and in slightly older children PTA are preferred.

The impedance audiometry is, of course, possible at any age. It can only however only tell us about the volume of the ear canal, compliance and middle ear pressure. What is more pertinent is to find out if the cochlear function and the sensorineural component is functioning normally or not. Therefore, PTA is vital.

2.20   Objective Audiological Assessment (Otoacoustic Emissions)

This test is routinely used across the NHS for neonatal screening for deafness. Its physiological basis is the fact that a healthy cochlea emits a faint response on exposure to a stimulus of sound. A clicking sound introduced through an ear piece containing a microphone and a speaker will pick up the response. Recording is made on a computer, confirming the presence of a normally functioning cochlea or a deficit requiring further investigations. However, it must be mentioned that a poor response may not necessarily mean deafness, as ambient noise in the background or middle ear effusion may make it difficult to record the faintness of responses.

2.21 Auditory Brain Response (ABR)

This is a very specialised test requiring sophisticated equipment and trained personnel. It is not performed on each and every child but only on those where we require to establish the nature of auditory pathway and the baby is too young for a behavioural test.

It may be used as screening test in the form of Automated Auditory Brainstem Response (AABR). The computer is commanded to pick up the response at the quiet sound levels.

More commonly ABR is employed for detailed evaluation of the auditory-brain pathway. The audiologist interprets the results of different sounds to which the child is exposed to stimulate the cochlea and the auditory nerve. The child may need to be sedated in some situations, as any disturbance may record artefacts.

2.22 Behavioural Tests

This is an intensive and fairly time-consuming testing procedure which is routinely performed in our audiology labs, as indeed in most audiology departments.

2.22.1 Visual Response Audiometry (VR)

This behavioural test is most suitable for hearing assessment in young infants between the ages of 6 months to about two and a half years. It involves a team of audiologists to check the response, in a soundproof audiosensitive, acoustically treated room. One audiologist plays the signals at variable frequencies through speakers. The other audiologist sitting by the child in the testing room notes the response. Every time the child turns the head to one side trying to locate the sound signal, he is rewarded with a musical toy. This test has a few limitations, as one can confirm the presence of hearing or otherwise at different levels of intensities and frequencies, but not be able to check each ear specifically.

2.22.2 Pure Tone Audiometry

It is routinely employed in all age groups, including the children above the age of 3 years to an elderly person of 80 plus. In children the audiologists employ such techniques which may make the child feel comfortable as if playing games. A common ploy used is that of 'men in the boat' or 'a peg on the board' etc. In adults, of course this is the commonest and most reliable tool for testing the hearing. It records the air conduction levels at different frequencies ranging from 250 to 8,000 Hz. The speech range is between 250 and 4,000 Hz. Any one who responds positively to this range should develop a normal speech, except if the child has a non-otological reason such as mental retardation or Global Developmental Delay.

The intensity of sound is changed by the audiologist from either the higher to lower levels or vice versa to establish the level of the patient's hearing. A cut-off point at 20 dB(A) is taken as a normal value. Bone conduction is recorded to establish the efficiency of the cochlea. In fact it is taught in most books that the bone conduction is the true representative of the nerve function and air conduction a true reflection of the middle and outer ear efficiency.

2.23   Speech Discrimination Audiometry

It is sometimes employed in children with delayed speech. The child's ability to hear and pick up specified table of words played from a recording is tested. The selected words cover most if not all frequencies that a normal person should be able to pick up in a given speech. The audiologist can deliver the words personally also at varying levels of volume and intensity to reward the child with a toy each time he repeats after the audiologist correctly. It is also used in assessing the sign language in some children.

References

Bender MB (1965) Oscillopsia. Arch Neurol 13(2):204–213

Cal R, Bahmad F Jr. (2009) Vestibular investigations. Revisat Braileira de Otlaringologica. 75(3):456–462, 1808–8686

Chiu CM, Huang SF, Tsai PY, Wang RY, Chuang TY, Sung WH (2010) Computer-aided vestibular auto rotational testing of the vestibulo-ocular reflex in senile vestibular dysfunction. Comput Methods Programs Biomed 97(1):92–98

Cohen HS, Kimball KT (2008) Usefulness of some current balance tests for identifying individuals with disequilibrium due to vestibular impairments. J Vestib Res 18(5–6):295–303, 0957–4271; 0957–4271

Crawford JD, Villis T (1991) Axes of eye rotation and Listing's law during the rotation of head. J Neurphysiol 65(3):407–423

Dell'Osso LF, Daroff RB (1999) Eye movement characteristics and recording techniques. In: Glaser JS (ed) Neuro-ophthalmology, pp 327–344

Hoffman RM, Einstadter D, Kroenke K (1999) Evaluating dizziness. Am J Med 107(5):468–478, 0002–9343

Donnellan K, Wei W, Jeffcoat B, Mustain W, Xu Y, Eby T, Phd WZ (2010) Frequency Tuning of BOVEMP recorded from extaraocular muscles in normal human subjects. Laryngoscope 120(12):2555–2560

King JE, Gonzalez JE, Fuller MI (2006) Development of a vestibular tasking device for use in vestibular assessment. J Vestib Res 16(1–2):57–67, 0957–4271

Korres S et al (2009) The diagnostic importance of electronystagmography and magnetic resonance imaging in vestibular disorders. J Laryngol Otol 123(8):851–856, 0022–2151;1748–5460

Lemajic-Komazec S, Komazec Z (2006) Initial evaluation of vertigo. Med Pregl 59(11–12):585–590, 0025–8105;0025–8105

MacDougall HG, Weber KP, McGarvie LA, Halmagyi GM, Curthoys IS (2009) The video head impulse test: diagnostic accuracy in peripheral vestibulopathy. Neurology 73(14):1134–1141, 0028–3878;1526–632X

Mudduwa R, Kara N, Whelan D, Banerjee A (2010) Vestibular evoked myogenic potentials: review. J Laryngol Otol 124:1043–1050

Paine M (2005) Dealing with dizziness. Aust Prescr 28:94–97

Philips JS, FitzGerald JE, Bath AP (2009) The role of vestibular assessment. J Otol Laryngol 123(11):1212–1250, 0022–2151; 1748–5460

Polensek SH, Sterk CE, Tusa RJ (2008) Screening for vestibular disorders: a study of clinicians' compliance with recommended practices. Med Sci Monit 14(5):CR238–CR242, 1234–1010; 1234–101

Rauch SD (2006) Vestibular evoked myogenic potentials. Curr Opin Otolaryngol Head Neck Surg 14(5):299–304, 1068–9508

Raymond J, Dememes D, Nieoullon A (1988) Neurotransmitters in vestibular pathways. In: Pompeiano O, Allum JHJ (eds) Vestibulospinal control of posture and locomotion, Prog Brain Res, Vol. 76. Montpellier and Marseille, France, pp 29–44

Sakakura K, Takahashi K, Takayasu Y, Chikamatsu K, Furuya N (2005) Novel method for recording vestibular evoked myogenic potential: minimally invasive recording on neck extensor muscles. Laryngoscope 115(10):1768–1773, 0023–852X

Sloane P, Blazer D, George L (1989) Dizziness in community elderly population. J Am Geitr Soc 37:101–108

Thabet E (2008) Evaluation of patients with acute vestibular syndrome. Euro Arch Otorhinolaryngol 265(3):341–349

Virk S, McConville KM (2006) Virtual realty applications in improving postural control and minimising falls. Med Biol Soc 1:2694–2697; 1557–170X

Vital D, Hegermann SC, Straumann D, Bergamin O, Bocklish CJ, Angehrn D, Schmitt KU, Probst R (2010) A new dynamic visual acuity test to assess peripheral vestibular function. Arch Otolaryngol Head Neck Surg 136(7):686–691, 0886–4470; 1538–36X

Whitney SL, Wrisley DM, Marchetti GF, Gee MA, Redfern MS, Furman JM (2005) Clinical measurement of sit-to-stand performance in people with balance disorders: validity of data for the Five-Times-Sit-to-Stand Test. Phys Ther 85(10):1034–1045, 0031–9023; 0031–9023

Yokota J, Imai H, Okuda O et al (1993) Inverted burns nystagmus in arachnoid cysts of the cerebellopontine angle. Eur Neurol 33:62

Further Reading

Hall JE, Guyton AC (2011) A text book of Physiology, 9th edn. W.B. Saunders, Philadelphia, p 724

Luxon L (ed) (2003) Text book of audiological medicine: clinical aspects of hearing and balance. Martin Dunitz/Taylor and Francis Group, London

Seikel JA, King DW, Drumright D (2009) Anatomy and physiology of Speech. Language and Hearing, 4th edn. San Diego, p 582

Martini F (1992) Fundamentals of Anatomy and Physiology, 2nd edn. Prentice-Hall, NJ, 07632

Part II

Clinical Conditions

Meniere's Disease

3

Meniere's disease is an important cause to remember. It is almost an icon for vertigo, a hallmark or a flag bearer. Its epidemiology, as described elsewhere in the first chapter, varies between different populations and different regions.

In the UK it is often considered to be an absolutely essential differential diagnosis in patients presenting with vertigo, tinnitus and hearing loss. Perhaps it may not be the first amongst its equals, as many other causes seem to offer it a fierce competition.

Vertigo caused by the labyrinthine instability has been recorded in the annals of history from ancient times. It is said that Julius Caesar suffered with it and surely many other historical figures before him. But not until 1861, the condition was christened, when Dr. Meniere an eminent French physician duly identified the relationship between the acute episodes of vertigo and the malfunctioning labyrinth in some of his patients. Therefore, the condition became associated with his name and has often been labelled a syndrome rather than a disease.

The exact aetiology of Meniere's disease remains unknown. Several hypotheses have been put forward over the years, but none has so far convincingly proved to be an absolute truth.

It is said that due to the vascular spasm in the cochlear artery, which is an end artery, the vascularity of stria vascularis becomes compromised resulting in abnormal physiological activity within the confines of the scala media. Either there is sudden and spontaneous overproduction of the endolymph or the decline in its absorption by the stria vascularis, resulting in accumulation of excessive quantities of this fluid within the narrow confines of the scala tympani. This in turn exerts pressure on the peripheral structures such as the organ of Corti, resulting in fluctuation of hearing during the attack and tinnitus which may have been present initially but becomes pronounced and extremely distressing. The patient also feels fullness of the ear for the same reason, and since the vestibular neuroepithelial tissue has close connexions with various pathways, e.g. the vestibulo-spinal and vestibulo-cerebellar tracts, the symptoms of volatile vertigo set in. Impulses may

S.H. Zaidi, A. Sinha, *Vertigo*,
DOI 10.1007/978-3-642-36485-3_3, © Springer-Verlag Berlin Heidelberg 2013

also be transmitted to the vagal nuclei sitting in close proximity, resulting in the production of vasovagal symptoms like nausea, sickness, sweating, palpitation, bradycardia and even syncope.

For a long time, scientist and clinicians have pondered over the possibility of it being an autoimmune disease. No conclusive evidence has been found in favour of this hypothesis.

More recently, attention has been focused on the immunological factors affecting the endolymphatic sac. Brenner et al. (2004) found that 25 % of their patients with Meniere's disease also suffered from autoimmune thyroid disease. We feel this study deserves due emphasis and perhaps more in death analysis. We have no data just yet to support a hypothesis of an autoimmune nature for Meniere's but would certainly look into it in the future, particularly in our head and neck clinics, where thyroid-related patients are seen on a weekly basis.

Ruckenstein (2002) studied the blood sample of 40 patients with unilateral Meniere's disease, for specific immunological values including CBC, ANA anti-Sjogren antibodies, RF, complement antiphospholipid antibodies, western blot for cardiac shock proteins, MHA and Lyme disease profiles. It was indeed an exhaustive research, based upon sound and thorough haematological investigations.

They concluded that it is highly unlikely that autoimmune aetiologies may play a significant role in their subjects of unilateral Meniere's disease. More studies are definitely required in this arena, as so far no conclusive etiological factor for Meniere's has been found. Autoimmune hypothesis certainly deserves due evaluation and further study. Meniere's is an old disease and many theories have been presented by masters over the years, without arriving at a consensus. Immunology is a growing field and many diseases, which were previously thought to be of infective (e.g. sarcoidosis), or non-specific origin, have turned out to be autoimmune. Meniere's certainly merits an enquiry on this ground. We would keenly look into this investigative research as a possible cause of Meniere's.

As mentioned elsewhere in this book, some of these patients may have a history of migraine. It is therefore a possibility that some underlying factors like diet, emotions, and stress may have a role to play in the causation of Meniere's disease. Besides, the two may have a common pathophysiology.

Typically, the patient is young and generally healthy. An aura of an impending disaster is noticed by the patient which could be felt as aural fullness or visual symptoms followed by a volatile attack of vertigo. It is nearly crippling and extremely frightening when it happens the first time ever. Tinnitus becomes pounding and unbearable fullness of the ear and fluctuation of hearing are noticed by the patient. Nausea, vomiting, pallor, sweating, etc. may or may not occur. The disease may begin in one ear and remain confined to only one side for a number of years, or it may affect both ears simultaneously. Silverstein (1989) believes that bilateral Meniere's is as low as 17 % though others have given the incidence of bilateral Meniere's up to 50 % of reported cases. His study is considered to be a pioneering study in this field.

The attack may last from a few minutes to several hours, even days. The fear of TIA, stroke, a heart attack or worse – a brain tumour instantly – crosses his mind.

Gradually, the symptoms settle down, and apart from slight to moderate degree of hearing loss and tinnitus, most symptoms disappear and the patient is immensely relieved.

The family doctor has no difficulty in diagnosing such a case and a short course of an anti-vertiginous drug or a similar labyrinthine sedative plus a word of reassurance are good enough for the patient to settled own. Obviously, the fear of life associated with the attack makes him request for a specialist referral, but it is advisable that a thorough investigation of such a case be carried out at the GP level before a referral. Many metabolic and some neurological conditions quite closely mimic Meniere's; hence, an experienced GP usually arranges for routine blood picture, glucose and lipids profile as indeed any serological tests if justified.

Urine analysis followed by a blood test for glucose metabolism may be the simplest tests that should exclude at least one major cause of fainting attacks, i.e. diabetes, and that is usually the routine in most family practices.

The specialist's role is secondary. Apart from a detailed history, a thorough clinical examination and an audiological profile, little else, are required in most cases. The history is so typical that the vestibular function tests may not always be required except in some atypical cases.

MRI is usually not required in Meniere's except in a vertiginous case of suspected acoustic neuroma or a demyelinising disorder such as MS. It is highly unusual, but both can sometimes coexist.

Kasai and colleagues (2009) see some justification in employing an MRI in Meniere's. They observed that an MRI after an intratympanic gadolinium injection can reveal endolymphatic hydrops in patients with delayed endolymphatic hydrops. They concur with the general practice that Meniere's is usually diagnosed with history, clinical findings, audiological and vestibular investigations. In their view an MRI seems to add a new dimension to the diagnostic arsenal.

It is a fine study that describes various intricacies of diagnostic imaging in the endolymphatic hydrops. An interesting suggestion though the cost versus benefits may be an issue in these days of limited resources. We believe that a clinical diagnosis in a classical case of Meniere's disease is simple, trustworthy and usually reliable. An MRI may certainly be considered if one suspects an additional pathology, which is rare, though possible. Coexistence of middle ear infection or a demyelinising disease is not a remote possibility. We tend to rely more upon our clinical diagnosis and save the adventitious tests for more complex issues.

Many physicians find acute vertigo a diagnostic challenge. Meniere's may have many differential diagnoses, although a typical case of Meniere's may hardly be missed.

Seemungal (2007) reviewed the evidence outlining the clinical presentation of acute, central and peripheral dizzy syndromes and suggested when clinicians may consider acute neuroimaging. The author noted that recent evidence highlights the difficulty that acute vertigo may sometimes pose to the clinician. For example, migrainous vertigo may have occulomotor abnormalities suggestive of either central neurological or peripheral vestibular dysfunction. Furthermore, vertebrobasilar stroke syndromes may mimic peripheral disorders such as vestibular neuritis, or when there is hearing involvement, Meniere's disease may come to mind.

It was thus summarised that despite the advancement, the assessment of acute vertigo has not become any easier for the non-specialist. Although the commonest causes are benign, serious conditions such as stroke may masquerade as a peripheral labyrinthine disorder, and conversely benign conditions such as migrainous vertigo may have clinical characteristics of central disorders. These findings re-emphasise the need for a comprehensive history and a thorough clinical evaluation of the acutely dizzy patient.

Chronological method of evaluating a case of vertigo was highlighted by Kerr (2005). He believes that the most important step in the diagnosis is an unhurried and detailed history, bearing in mind that many patients will have difficulty in describing their symptoms. A detailed neurological examination is usually unnecessary, but one must examine the ears and the cranial nerves, check for any evidence for defective function of the cerebellum and the locomotor system, and look for the presence of nystagmus. The common error of carrying out investigations in place of a detailed history is to be avoided. In many cases, investigations are not required at all, although it is the author's practice to do a routine pure tone audiogram with basic assessment of speech discrimination. Quite rightly Kerr points out that there is no indication for routine caloric testing, imaging or blood analysis, each of which should be carried out only when there are specific indications. And he agrees with all other clinicians in the statement that it is only in exceptional situations that specialised vestibular testing is required.

A clinician must be patient in listening to the patient, with an odd probing question. He is bound to be rewarded with some clues to the possible cause of patient's dizziness. Brief history and a hurried examination may miss out the minute foot marks, which are sometimes extremely valuable in catching a thief. In other words, one has to play the role of a sleuth and he will find joy at the end of his sojourn. Many physicians believe in leaving the diagnosis to a lab test. That regrettably kills the fine art of medicine, of employing our grey cells to sift through the mass of evidence, at the cost of depriving many patients of so many services due to the shortage of funds. Though claimed by all the gate keepers that they practice distributive justice, but do they indeed?

Case Report
P was born in March 1933 and presented with spells of rotatory vertigo with associated nausea about 15 years ago. She described being unable to walk in a starlight line and had to remain in bed for a few days feeling unwell for a period of about 2–3 weeks. Her hearing apparently deteriorated for 2–3 days, and she felt that sounds felt distorted when the hearing returned initially. She said that her hearing loss in the left ear began at that time. She also described having undergone tests for her dizziness, which sounded like calorimetry, following which she was told that she suffered with Meniere's disease.

P said that she did not experience any rotatory vertigo or being bedridden since her initial attack 15 years ago. She, however, said that she used to experience spells of imbalance two or three times a year. She was prescribed SERC, which she stopped taking about 6 years ago. Since then she took diuretic tablet and felt symptom-free for the last 4–5 years until August/September 2009. At this time she felt off balance and almost as if drunk, upon waking up in the morning. The feeling lasted for 3 days. She also noticed reduction in her hearing lasting a day followed by distortion of sounds. In between the attacks P experienced light-headedness on bending down and upon standing up. She reported that 2 years ago she had turned her head quickly which had led to her fall. She said that she is currently leading a normal life and doing her daily chores without a problem.

The patient denied tinnitus, though she noticed a feeling of constant pressure in her left ear without noticing any change in this feeling during the spells of imbalance. The patient also told that she had a mastoid operation done upon her as a baby (which could have been drainage of an abscess or a cortical mastoidectomy, though the scar was imperceptible on inspection).

This patient also suffered with migraines as a teenager causing her severe headaches and dizziness. She also sustained an attack of angina 30 years ago and suffered with hypothyroidism. Therefore, she was on thyroxin, a benzoflouride and a beta blocker. P also suffered with cervical arthritis without causing any noticeable restriction of her neck movements.

Routine otoscopy revealed no abnormalities. The tympanometry indicated normal middle ear function bilaterally. Pure tone audiometry showed a moderate degree of sensorineural hearing loss confined to the higher frequencies in the right ear and a similar loss involving all the frequencies on the left side. Slight improvement was noted at 250 K on the left side compared to an audiogram recorded 4 months earlier.

On functional testing, this patient was unable to maintain her balance with reduced visual and proprioceptive inputs. Ocular motor testing using VNG revealed no spontaneous or rebound nystagmus. Upon gaze testing without fixation, a low-level right-beating nystagmus was noticed, with eyes directed to the right and a low-level left-beating nystagmus with eyes directed to the left. This may, however, have been an end point nystagmus as she had difficulty keeping her eyes in the correct position. Testing of random saccades and smooth pursuit showed no abnormalities. Calorimetry was not undertaken due to the history of unstable angina.

The results of vestibular tests, therefore, did not suggest any central or peripheral vestibular lesion. A fresh calorimetry would have been of immense help but was contraindicated. Elements of P's history and the slight change in her hearing on the left side were in keeping with Meniere's disease, which was diagnosed in her many years ago when she apparently had undergone calorimetry also.

She was advised to return to the outpatient clinic for a follow-up.

Case Report

P was born in 1941 and was seen in our vestibular lab for detailed assessments in April 2010. She reported two episodes of recent bouts of dizziness, which she described as rotatory in nature initiated by her turning her head in bed. She also reported the onset of similar, more marked, symptoms in January 2010 when undergoing exercises given by her GP that involved head turns. There was no associated nausea during the previous episodes. She however said that she had sensation of 'heaviness' in her left ear, reduction in hearing in her left ear and an exacerbation of her long-standing left-sided tinnitus. In the week leading up to the episodes of dizziness at least on two previous occasion in September 2009 and January 2010, she mentioned that gaze fixation helped to alleviate her symptoms during spell, and she had tendency to guard against getting out of bed too quickly for the fear of provoking her symptoms, although it had been less frequent since November.

P also reported an episode of rotatory vertigo in 1997; the symptoms of which lasted half a day and caused her to stagger when she tried to walk. She said she was unwell at the time and had no associated nausea or variation in her hearing or indeed tinnitus. She, however, noticed heaviness in her left ear during the spell but said that she also had trigeminal neuralgia at the time, though it was diagnosed a few years later in 2005.

P reported a fluctuating, left-sided gradual deterioration in her hearing over the last 3–4 years. She also reported a continuous 'buzzing' left-sided tinnitus, more pronounced when alone. She also noticed a decline in her hearing and increased heaviness in her left ear at that time. She also received medication for her coronary heart disease.

Otoscopy was normal bilaterally. Tympanometry was fine on each side too, with ipsilateral acoustic reflexes showing normal recordings on each side. Pure tone audiometry showed normal hearing levels on the right side with the exception of 25 dbHL threshold at 8 kHz and a mild sensorineural hearing loss on the left side. Deterioration in hearing thresholds was noted compared with the tests recorded in March 2008.

Upon functional testing, P was able to maintain her balance with reduced visual and proprioceptive inputs. Ocular motor testing using VNG revealed no spontaneous, gaze-evoked or rebound nystagmus. No abnormalities were detected upon testing of random saccades or smooth pursuit. Dix–Hallpike testing was negative bilaterally. Monothermal screening caloric test using warm water produced robust and approximately equal responses bilaterally. Visual fixation index was normal.

It was therefore inferred that P had Meniere's disease with a possibility of fluctuating vestibular functions. It was also considered a possibility that P also had suffered with BPPV which had resolved spontaneously.

Case Report

P was born in 1940 and presented with a history of an ear infection in his right ear a year ago followed by imbalance until now. He also noticed light-headedness on standing up from a sitting posture or indeed on moving around. He felt that he may fall down while walking up the stairs.

No abnormalities were noted on otoscopy with normal tympanometry bilaterally. Ocular motor testing revealed no significant spontaneous, gaze-evoked or rebound nystagmus. No abnormalities of saccadic eye movements were detected either. P continually jumped his eyes on smooth pursuit; this may have been due to failure to fully comprehend the test and its motives. Standard calorimetry revealed a significant canal paresis on the right side, with significant directional preponderance to the left.

It was therefore concluded from the results that a significant peripheral vestibular weakness existed on the right side. Poor smooth pursuit could well be a central sign but can also be caused by lack of attention or failure to concentrate. P was advised to commence Cawthorne–Cooksey exercise with a follow-up appointment to monitor his progress.

Case Report

P born in 1979 was seen in the vestibular lab in Feb 2010, with a history of imbalance for the last 3 months. She described her symptoms to appear spontaneously in the middle of the night with a sensation of vertigo and vomiting. The sensation continued for a couple of weeks. It then reduced to daily spells noticed upon movement only and further reduced to similar episodes noticed only four to five times in a week. She describes her feeling akin to 'being on the waltz', though it was paroxysmal, spontaneous and repetitive.

P wore hearing aids bilaterally and said that her hearing loss that began about 18 months ago had deteriorated gradually over the last few months. She had no familial history of deafness or hearing impairment and suffered with occasional tinnitus worse on the right side. She had frequent headaches, along with migraine and visual disturbances. P also suffered from asthma, fibromyalgia and epilepsy and had Ehlers–Danlos syndrome.

Ocular motor testing using videonystagmography revealed no spontaneous, rebound or gaze-evoked nystagmus. No abnormalities of smooth pursuit were detected. Saccadic eye movements had prolonged latency in both right and left directions. Accuracy and velocity of saccade were within the normal limits to the left but borderline to the right. The Dix–Hallpike testing was negative bilaterally. Calorimetry was contraindicated on account of her epilepsy. The head shake test provoked a right-beating nystagmus. The head thrust test was bilaterally negative.

It was therefore concluded that a peripheral vestibular lesion was a strong possibility of Meniere's disease. The abnormal saccades might suggest a central lesion; however, 'normal range' of saccadic parameters is thought to be different in epileptic patients.

P was commenced on Cawthorne–Cooksey exercises to help her with her peripheral vestibular lesion.

Case Report

P born in 1944 presented with short spells of rotatory vertigo when turning to her left in her bed and when dorsiflexing or extending her head and neck. These spells lasted between 10 and 15 s and occurred approximately every 3 or 4 days. Sometimes she also had accompanying nausea. The initial attack happened about a year ago when she had a prolonged dizzy spells, feeling almost like a drunk, accompanied by nausea and vomiting. She also mentioned that in between the attacks she 'never felt quite right'. She also had a tendency to veer to the left on walking. She also found it hard to drive her mobility car, thus limiting her ability significantly to go out and about, adversely affecting her quality of life.

She had been wearing hearing aid since last 6 years. She reported that her hearing sometimes drops on the right side without any known reason. She suspected it to be due to a faulty hearing aid. She did not notice any association between her dizzy spells and the fall in her hearing levels nor did she notice any pressure feelings in her ears. She only had occasional tinnitus, which was not bothersome. In the past she suffered with migraines which gradually resolved. She occasionally had mild headaches flashing in her eyes. She also suffered from bodily arthritis restricting her movements. Besides, she was a chronic renal patient and had coronary artery stented a few years ago.

Her otoscopy was normal with normal compliance and middle ear pressure on the left but some evidence of Eustachian tube dysfunction on the right side. PTA showed bilateral high-frequency sensorineural hearing loss, which had not worsened since the last recorded audiogram 6 years ago.

Using the videonystagmography, the occulomotor nerve testing revealed no spontaneous or rebound nystagmus and no abnormalities of smooth pursuit or random saccades. The right-beating nystagmus (4.2 %) was observed when she was gazing to the right without fixation but at no other gaze direction. The Dix–Hallpike manoeuvre was contraindicated due to her arthritis. Calorimetry was also contraindicated to her compromised heart condition.

Unfortunately, only a few tests could be carried out on this patient, though the gaze test results indicated peripheral lesion. Cawthorne–Cooksey exercise was commenced and a follow-up appointment was arranged.

Case Report

P was seen in the vestibular lab in March 2010 with a history of an acute episode of volatile vertigo experienced about 4 months ago. She experienced 10–20 s of oscillopsia but did not note any rotation. She had nausea and vomiting for 2 days. She was able to walk about but initially bumped into objects around her. Since her vertiginous episode, P has felt sensation of being 'pushed down'. The feeling worsened on looking down to the floor on sudden movement of head. She suspected that she may veer to right and had noticed that rolling over on her right side made her symptoms worse. She took Stemetil after the initial episode but soon stopped it and took betahistine for 3 weeks with guarded benefit.

P was an informed and knowledgeable patient who noticed a fall in her hearing in her right ear since her episode of imbalance. She also had bilateral high-pitched tinnitus 2 days after the episode. This was now constant and more noticeable in a quiet surrounding. There was no history of ear infection, though she had suffered with migraine and photophobia, without dizziness.

The otoscopy was normal. PTA showed an island of mild hearing loss at 1 kHz in the right ear, with a normal tympanogram.

P was able to maintain balance with reduced visual and proprioceptive inputs. Ocular motor testing using VNG revealed no spontaneous, gaze-evoked or rebound nystagmus. Persistent horizontal eye movements were recorded on gaze testing without fixation to the right and left, but there was no nystagmus. No abnormalities were recorded on testing of random saccades or smooth pursuits at 0.45 Hz. Dix–Hallpike test produced no nystagmus or subjective sensation on the right or the left side. Calorimetry was arranged on later date. It was however concluded that P could have a unilateral labyrinthine lesion. She was commenced upon Cawthorne–Cooksey exercises, pending calorimetry and a follow-up.

Meniere's disease is usually unilateral and may sometimes pose a diagnostic problem, particularly if it does not have the typical presenting features, and yet calorimetry may show unilateral canal preponderance or a hypofunction. Such cases may require further vestibular investigations.

Unilateral vestibular hypofunction was evaluated as a clinical entity contributing towards the menace of vertigo by Schonfeld and colleagues (2010).

Their findings demonstrated that an enduring unilateral utricular dysfunction, possibly together with canal hypofunction, can occur after labyrinthine disease or injury. They also suggested that unilateral, isolated utricular dysfunction – or utricle paresis – can occur, representing a novel entity in the differential diagnosis of peripheral vestibular function.

It is worth noting that the term 'utricular paresis' is an innovative term, and we may witness its application more often in the future.

Migraine is definitely known to diminish in intensity, severity and frequency with age. Meniere's disease is suspected to have a similar pathophysiology by some workers as discussed elsewhere in this book. Does Meniere's behave similarly? Well, Huppert et al. (2010) audited the long-term picture of Meniere's disease. They analysed 46 studies, in which a total of 7,852 had been evaluated. They discovered that the frequency of attacks of vertigo diminished with the passage of time over a period of 5–10 years. They also made a note that the hearing loss varying between 50 and 60 dB and vestibular dysfunction of about 35–50 % occurred during the initial few years. As is generally the observation, Huppert et al. reaffirm that spontaneous remission is common. They also noted that the drop attacks may occur early or late in the course of the disease. Furthermore, bilateral involvement increases with the duration, i.e. longevity of disease. In their practice, they noted that up to 35 % would show involvement of both ears within 10 years, rising up to 47 % in couple of decades. This is a very informative and comprehensive study, which gives us a lot of information about the impact of time and duration upon Meniere's disease. Further studies are certainly required to confirm the hypothesis that Meniere's does diminish in its intensity with age.

Numerous diagnostic tests are available for evaluation of vertigo. VEMP is gaining rapid promotion amongst the battery of such tests, especially in rather unusual clinical scenarios. Timmer et al. (2006) found that VEMP thresholds were more often elevated or absent in patients with Meniere's disease experiencing Tumarkin drop attacks than in those without. It was concluded in this retrospective study that advanced disease involving the saccule was responsible for the Tumarkin drop attacks. VEMP may indeed be a clinically valuable metric for measuring the severity of the disease or its further progress. It could well prove to be an indicator towards the long-term prognosis of the disease and may be employed to warn against the future drop attacks, so very disturbing and often demoralising to an unwarned patient.

The value of VEMP in pinpointing the exact location of pathology is proving to be an important breakthrough. It is an exciting fact that one can narrow down the search even further. Tumarkin phenomenon, fortunately, is not so common, but it is good to learn that it can now be traced right up to its origins as far as the causative elements are concerned.

Tumarkin phenomenon is also called the 'otolith crisis of Tumarkin'. He described this condition in 1936 (Ruckenstein et al. 2002), attributing it to spontaneous mechanical deformation of the otolith organs, i.e. utricle and saccule, resulting in a rapid, sudden and alarming activation of the vestibular reflexes. These drop attacks may require repositioning of the otolith particles.

Iwasaki et al. (2005) looked at the value of VEMP in the diagnosis of Meniere's. They observed that the combined use of vestibular-evoked myogenic potential (VEMP) and calorimetry enabled them to examine the function of the inferior and superior vestibular nerves separately. They noted that although results of VEMP testing and caloric response testing have been reported for many diseases, a clinical entity showing abnormal VEMP responses but normal caloric test responses has rarely been reported. The aim of their study was to investigate the clinical features of diseases showing abnormal VEMP responses with normal caloric test responses. This study of more than 800 dizzy patients concluded that apart from Meniere's disease, acoustic neuroma and sudden deafness with vertigo, which are already known as diseases with abnormal VEMP responses but normal caloric test responses, some patients might be diagnosed as having a disease that involves only the inferior vestibular nerve region. It goes without saying that vestibular investigations have opened new vista in the field of diagnostics and precision of the site of malfunction.

The role of VEMP as a new and extremely helpful tool in the diagnosis of vestibular vertigo is duly highlighted by this study.

Prepageran and colleagues (2005) described an interesting clinical scenario supplemented with contemporary diagnostic tools. They believe that symptomatic high-frequency/acceleration vestibular loss is a distinct clinical entity that can be missed on conventional ENG with caloric testing. They advise that under certain circumstances, symptomatic patients with a high-frequency/acceleration vestibular loss should undergo a magnetic scleral search coil (MSSC) study for confirmation, if required.

They believe that normal electronystagmography (ENG) with conventional calorimetry is inadequate for diagnosing clinically significant high-frequency/acceleration vestibular loss. Therefore, they investigated the patients with persistent peripheral vestibular dysfunction despite normal conventional calorimetry on ENG, who underwent high-frequency/acceleration horizontal magnetic scleral search coil (MSSC) eye movement studies. Then they reviewed the clinical findings and results from audiometric tests, conventional ENG with conventional calorimetry and MSSC tests. They believe that ENG caloric testing evaluates the function of the lateral semicircular canal and should be considered a non-physiological test primarily of low-frequency vestibular function. High-frequency/acceleration head thrust testing clinically detected a 'high-frequency/acceleration vestibular loss' in 72.7 % of the cases. Their study recommends the employment of the latter technique more frequently. Obviously, it is more of a research tool to be employed under special circumstances and in dedicated places, such as the balance clinics which must be amply supported with the necessary diagnostic tools and trained staff. In a busy ENT clinic, such diagnostic tools are rarely employed, though ideally they should be, as the vertiginous cause can be literarily pinpointed through such measures.

Routine conventional and traditional methods of vestibular investigation compared with an ENG have been the topic of much debate in some circles. Arriaga and colleagues (2005) investigated the sensitivity of rotational chair (ROTO) with electronystagmography in peripheral vestibular pathology. After an exhaustive study, they concluded that ROTO was indeed a more sensitive diagnostic study of peripheral vestibular pathology. They opined that the higher sensitivity of ROTO compared with ENG may support its employment as the primary means of diagnostic evaluation. We employ ROTO in selected few paediatric cases, and our experience is certainly not as vast as them. ENG, in their view, on the other hand, is not an investigation of choice anymore, as it has been all but replaced by VNG.

We employ VNGs in our lab as a standard investigation in those cases that justify detailed analysis, such as Meniere's or a suspected central pathology.

It is such an invaluable tool in the diagnostic arsenal of our services that we have allocated it a separate chapter. For want of space and other constraints, only a few representative VNGs are included in this book (Fig. 2.5) under the chapter labelled as VNGs (Chap. 2).

Calorimetry has stood the test of time as it remains the touchstone of vestibular diagnostics. We trust it thoroughly and our vestibular colleagues employ it when required except when there may be a contraindication such as an unstable angina or uncontrolled hypertension. And that is for the fear that calorimetry may potentiate a vasovagal collapse. Calorimetry is however being challenged by vHIT, but time alone will tell.

Palomar-Asenjo (2006) investigated the hypothesis if an association existed between the parameters of calorimetry and rotatory chair tests in patients with unilateral Meniere's disease. They subjected 100 patients with unilateral Meniere's disease to these tests, including sinusoidal harmonic acceleration and impulsive tests, on the same day.

Essential and common variables such as the canal paresis and directional preponderance were assessed in calorimetry. Then different variables were measured in the rotatory chair test based on the existence of abnormal parameters in the vestibulo-ocular reflex at two or three consecutive frequencies of those tested and on the time constant of the vestibulo-ocular reflex.

The study found out that an abnormal result in the caloric test was obtained in 73 % of the patients. In the rotatory chair test, the most frequent abnormal findings involved increases in the normal phase lead at two consecutive frequencies tested (23 %). There was a stronger association between an abnormal result in phase, gain and/or symmetry at three adjacent frequencies and a pathological result in the caloric test.

It was therefore concluded that very few of the criteria used to define the caloric and rotatory chair tests seem to be associated. This study confirmed the previous knowledge that both tests examine vestibulo-ocular reflex by different ways. Only when vestibular dysfunction is severe enough to show an abnormal result in at least three consecutive frequencies in the rotatory chair test, the caloric test is also found to be abnormal. Suffice it to say that both conventional calorimetry and the rotational vestibulometry are quite potent tools for assessment of the peripheral vestibular pathologies.

Acute sensorineural hearing loss has often been the cause of much concern in many cases. The exact aetiology remains doubtful in most situations, though any cause from a viral infection to ischemic changes has been incriminated.

Most of such patients are seen by the family physicians, but some may report to the emergency ENT services. The experience is absolutely frightening to the patient. The possibility of never regaining the hearing back to normal level is real, but this news must be carefully broken to an already-worried patient. An absolutely essential attribute for a physician to possess is the art of communication. Bad news needs a controlled, self-assured and gentle approach. Empathy and not sympathy are

required in such situations. Most medical curricula these days teach the communication skills to their undergraduates. It is absolutely necessary, in this day and age
of litigious culture.

Sudden deafness is usually unilateral but can be bilateral. The exact cause cannot
be established, though in a unilateral case viral exanthemata like mumps have often
been found guilty. Many audiologists and otologists would blame a sudden ischaemic in the cochlear artery, an end artery, to be the cause. Why does that happen, one
does not know. It is postulated that it could be a histamine-related event causing
spontaneous spasm, hence ischaemia of stria vascularis. Others believe that it could
well be a viral infection of an unknown nature. Steroid therapy introduced in ade-
quate quantities and at an appropriate time may limit the damage. Not always, but
many a times, vertigo may be associated with an acute deafness.

Meniere's has often been considered as a differential diagnosis, particularly if
the loss is either profound or near total. Studies have been carried out on this subject
too. In one such study, Chen and Young evaluated the problem: Chen and Young
(2006). They pointed out that most patients with Meniere's disease reveal abnormal
vestibular-evoked myogenic potentials (VEMPs) with the recruitment phenomenon,
whereas most patients with sudden deafness display normal VEMPs without the
recruitment phenomenon. The purpose of their study was to recommend a diagnostic algorithm to differentiate between Meniere's and sudden deafness as the cause of
acute hearing loss. After a battery of well-designed tests for this study, Chen and
Young concluded and recommended using both the recruitment phenomenon and
VEMP testing as a diagnostic algorithm to differentiate between Meniere's diseases
and sudden deafness as the cause of acute hearing loss.

Surely, there is more to come in the field of diagnostics, not just for the Meniere's
but all other potential culprits.

And now let us discuss the treatment of Meniere's disease.

The treatment for Meniere's begins at the family physician's level. Sometimes
the patient may not be able to see the GP such as at a weekend or a holiday season
and the A& E or an urgent care centre becomes his first port of call.

Reassurance is the fundamental brick in the management of Meniere's. The
patient is so frightened that some have been known to call their solicitors for updat-
ing their will. Once it has been clarified that he does not have any life-threatening or
indeed disabling condition, one can see the relief in his attitude. Immediate treatment is either parenteral introduction of prochlorperazine (Stemetil) or Dramamine
or cinnarizine. Oral therapy should be discontinued as soon as the symptoms
improve, and vestibular compensatory mechanisms must be given a chance to take
over the function of the damaged labyrinth.

A common remedy is the prescription of betahistine, which has been in vogue
since the last four decades or more and continues to enjoy the favour of both the family doctor and the specialist. It certainly has some advantages in preventing the attack
and, hence, should be prescribed as a prophylactic drug. Its dose is gradually adjusted
over a period of time lasting between a few weeks to a couple of months or less.
Once again, it is worth mentioning that the compensatory vestibular mechanism
should not be compromised with either a prophylactic or a therapeutic medicinal

treatment. That does not mean that one should wait and do nothing while the patient suffers. That is where the importance of clinical judgment comes in and that can neither be replaced by any technology nor indeed by any doctrine.

Karapolat et al. (2010) investigated the effect of high-dose betahistine treatment combined with vestibular rehabilitation on the disability, balance and postural stability in patients with unilateral vestibular disorder. They found out that both vestibular rehab (VR) and betahistine have a positive effect upon disability and imbalance in patients with unilateral vestibular disorder, but when betahistine was added to the rehab therapy, the postural stability was more effectively restored.

It is a well-known observation that vestibular rehabilitation has a positive effect on most cases of vertigo. Drugs are known to prevent recurrence and relief from repeated attacks of Meniere's, but prolonged use of drugs should be avoided as it slows down the natural vestibular compensatory mechanisms. It seems that a combination of short-duration medical treatment with rehabilitation therapy gives a better outcome.

In our practice we have found the combination to supersede the solitary form of treatment, i.e. with either the medicines or just the vestibular rehabilitation.

Surgical treatment of Meniere's disease has always been controversial. Meniere's disease is basically a metabolic disorder. It is best treated medically. However, surgery for vertigo has been in vogue since the last several decades. There was a time in late 1960s and early 1970s that several maestros like Howard and William House of the House Ear Institute California, Brackman, Silverstein, Fisch, Sheehy, Shea, Portmann Causse, Paparella, Tos, Mawson, Smyth and several other illustrious names excelled in the fine art of ear surgery and promoted their techniques through their institutions. The legend has it that one of the astronauts to land on the moon had undergone a shunt operation, thus making his flight to the moon and safe return to the lowly but lovely earth possible!

The fundamental principle underlying surgery for Meniere's is based upon the hypothesis that the symptoms are brought about by accumulation of excessive quantities of endolymph in the scala tympani, possibility due to either fibrosis or mechanical obstruction at the terminal end of the endolymphatic duct, discouraging the free flow and drainage of the endolymph into the subarachnoid space. One could, therefore, either decompress the saccus endolymphaticus or introduce a shunt between the endolymphatic duct and the subarachnoid space. The former was called the decompression procedure and the latter a shunt operation. Both groups had their promoters and supporters. For a couple of decades, surgery for Meniere's was a highly specialised field. Only a few centres and chosen few surgeons actually practised them.

Silverstein et al. (1989) studied the various modalities of surgical interventions and their long-term outcomes. The surgical procedures investigated were endolymphatic subarachnoid shunt (ELS), retrolabyrinthine neurectomy, middle fossa vestibular neurectomy and transmetal cochlear vestibular neurectomy. This substantial and highly influential study was carried out between 1974 and 1983. He found out that the spontaneous cure rate amongst the control group, i.e. nonsurgical patients, was 51 % after 2 years and 7 1 % after 3 or more years. The cure rate after ELS was

40 % after 2 years and 71 % after 3 or more years. So it was not statistically significant from the nonsurgical group. Silverstein discusses other results also in this study which was very comprehensive concluding that ELS did not improve control remission of vertigo in Meniere's.

Long-term intervals of remission are well documented in the course of Meniere's disease. It sometimes gives false hopes of total recovery from illness. Alas, the symptoms may reoccur with vengeance.

There are some interesting techniques which may or may not work but have their supporters. For instance, grommet insertion was practised and continues to be practised even today. As to how does it decompress the bulging endolymphatic space is difficult to explain, but it seems to work at least in some patients. It has been quite beneficial in a few of our patients also. It is possible that it may have a placebo effect as the opponents would argue, or perhaps the procedure may have coincided with a period of remission, which is not uncommon in Meniere's disease. Anyway, it certainly works in some patients!

In order to confirm the success or failure of a surgical intervention in the management of Meniere's, different tests can be employed. Calorimetry continues to enjoy much popularity despite a lapse of several decades since it was first introduced. As a matter of fact, it is still the touch stone of vestibulometry, as was highlighted by the following study.

Ulubil et al. (2008) evaluated the effect of endolymphatic sac surgery on vestibular functions using caloric testing and electronystagmography in more than 20 patients through their medical records. It was more like an audit than a descriptive analysis. They employed the ENG and recorded the absolute value of the caloric response of the operated ear and the degree of reduced vestibular response (RVR) rates as indicators of caloric functions which were then compared before and after surgery. After a comprehensive evaluation of the variables mentioned above, it was concluded that the endolymphatic sac surgery did not appear to be a vestibular destructive procedure. Therefore, it could be considered as a therapeutic alternative for patients with bilateral Meniere's disease who may have failed conservative management.

In the early 1970s, a renowned surgeon in Italy even promoted the unique and rather perplexing idea of depositing salt crystals of microscopic proportions in the region of round window through a tympanotomy. His null hypothesis being that salt being hygroscopic by nature would, through osmosis, create a biochemical gradient in the endolymphatic space, thus reducing the pressure resulting in the relief of symptoms. This practice did not gain much popularity. This illustration truly reflects the nature of enthusiasm that Meniere's created in those hay days of ear surgery.

Vestibular nerve section was practised by some neuro-otologists with guarded success. The procedure carried a high risk of co-morbidity, hence remained confined to very few centres. It never became popular.

Many studies have, however, been carried out which highlight the importance of vestibular neurectomy in intractable and uncontrollable Meniere's disease. One such study mentions that 80–85 % of patients according to world literature would show marked improvement in symptoms. Leveque et al. (2010) carried out a study to evaluate if vestibular neurectomy could indeed provide so much relief as mentioned elsewhere. They studied 24 patients 1 year after they underwent vestibular neurectomy through a retro-sigmoid approach. They performed a battery of tests including the kinetic test as well as the calorimetry. It was noted that postoperatively these patients showed areflexia on the operated side. Their study thus duly showed that the vestibular neurectomy can provide a complete vestibular deafferentation. One must however warrant the reader that it is a highly selective form of surgery possible in dedicated centres only. It has not gained much popularity over the years, especially because the practice of surgery has become highly defensive. Besides, the results may not be very exciting either.

Destruction of the affected labyrinth through what is called a total labyrinthectomy is yet another way of overcoming chronic unrelenting attacks of giddiness. It is applicable only to the cases with extremely poor hearing. Membranous labyrinthectomy gives relief from vertigo but also destroys the hearing. Furthermore, post-surgical rehabilitation through Cawthorne–Cooksey exercises is a lengthy process with a demanding schedule.

Deliberate destruction of the affected labyrinth can also be achieved with the use of ototoxic drugs like the aminoglycosides such as gentamicin injected into the ear. It offers satisfactory results, but it destroys the hearing and has therefore limited application to those cases only, where the disease has adversely affected the hearing. We have been successful in employing this method in several cases of chronic intractable Meniere's disease with severe to profound hearing impairment. The results have been positive and we would certainly recommend it in a selected number of cases who fail the medical treatment and have extremely poor hearing.

Bilateral selective labyrinthectomy is carried out in a few cases, but for obvious reasons, its application remains confined to those with near total or total loss of hearing along with an intractable, persistent, incurable and crippling vertigo.

Meniere's disease may go into hibernation and may not trouble the patient for variable lengths of time. It is also a self-limiting condition. Thus, its course varies between acute, repeated attacks almost debilitating a patient to rare and fleeting momentary bouts.

The pattern of Meniere's varies amongst the nations. Many factors such as age, stress and socio-economy seem to influence the overall picture. Japan is currently inundated with the ageing population. Some of whom suffer with vertigo caused by Meniere's.

Shojaku et al. (2009) investigated the incidence of new cases of Meniere's disease in 60-year-old subjects. They found it to have increased over time after correction for age distribution in the overall population. Fatigue and professional stress may have contributed in the recent increase in elderly-onset cases. It is an established fact that physical and mental fatigue can induce an onset of the disease. Clear changes were seen over time in the population-adjusted sex distribution of the disease and population-adjusted age at onset. According to this study, the number of definite cases in females versus males also increased. The proportion of cases in which onset occurred at 60 years of age or more increased over time when the number of cases in each age group was adjusted for changes in age distribution of the population over time. From the time of the third survey, there was a slight increase in the proportion of cases with bilateral involvement. The importance of such studies can hardly be emphasised enough, as the world is growing grey, and the burden of disease caused by Meniere's disease, as calculated by QALYS, is quite significant upon the economies. Detailed statistical data on the magnitude of a given condition can help the health economists plan even better.

Meniere's is a chronic intermittent, relapsing, condition with uncertainties and false sense of relief, leading to the risk of developing health anxiety. It is known to cause anxiety, depression, disability, adjustment disorders and dissociative disorders. Yardley and Kirby (2008) have discussed this issue in a paper, duly highlighting the insecurity of future attacks, leading the sufferers of a certain age to become housebound, avoiding going out unless with someone accompanied.

3.1   Lermoyez's Syndrome

This is an extremely rare cause of vertigo. As a matter of fact, it is usually confused with Meniere's disease, as the symptoms mimic closely. The only difference between Lermoyez's and Meniere's is in the reversal of symptoms. In the words of Lermoyez, the attack begins with 'numbness, goes deaf, and buzzes. Gradually the deafness becomes complete, when suddenly violent vertigo develops, and the hearing reappears (Baillie 1956). Clinically, it is noted that a patient with Lermoyez's feels nausea and sickness more acutely, which seem to relieve his symptoms.

Portmann, the legendary otologists of Bordeaux, France, described the pathophysiology of Lermoyez's as a condition akin to Raynaud 's phenomenon, involving the Cochlear artery, going into a sudden spasm, leading to the symptoms, followed by release of spasm and recovery (Baillie 1956). We must remember that the cochlear artery is an end artery with no collateral support. Its spasm is not a matter of ordinary significance. If the spasm does not improve, the artery may go into irrecoverable ischaemic, leading to loss of the inner ear function.

The reasons for a sudden spasm of the cochlear artery remain undetermined. As usual histamine release, or release of certain hitherto unidentified chemical mediators may be given the blame. Why does the spasm disappear? Well, obviously the same old presumption that the release of the chemical mediators stops and the already-secreted elements become gradually diluted, resulting in the reversal of symptoms.

References

Arriaga MA, Chen DA, Cenci KA (2005) Rotational chair (ROTO) instead of electronystagmography (ENG) as the primary vestibular test. Otolaryngol Head Neck Surg 133(3):329–333, 0194–5998; 0194–5998

Baillie WR (1956) Lermoyez syndrome. J Laryngol Otol 70:97–116

Brenner M, Hoistad D, Hain TC (2004) Prevalence of thyroid function in patients with Ménière's disease. Arch Otolaryngol Head Neck Surg 130(2):226–228

Chen CN, Young YH (2006) Differentiating the cause of acute sensorineural hearing loss between Meniere's disease and sudden deafness. Acta Otolaryngol 126(1):25–31, 0001–6489; 0001–6489

Huppert D, Strupp M, Brandt T (2010) Long term course of Meniere's revisited. Acta Otolaryngol 130(6):644–651, 0001–6489; 1651–2251

Iwasaki S, Takai Y, Ito K, Murofushi T (2005) Abnormal vestibular evoked myogenic potentials in the presence of normal caloric responses. Otol Neurotol 26(6):1196–1199, 1531–7129; 1531–7129

Karapolat H, Celebisoy N, Kirzali Y, Bilgen C, Eyigor S, Gode S, Akyuz A, Kirzali T (2010) Does Beatstine treatment have additional benefits to vestibular rehabilitation. Eur Arch Otorhinolaryngol 267(8):1207–1212, 0937–4477.16/6

Kasai S, Teranishi M, Katayama N, Sugiura M, Nakata S, Sone M, Naganawa S, Nakashima T (2009) Endolymphatic space imaging in patients with delayed endolymphatic hydrops. Acta Otolaryngol 129(11):1169–1174, 0001–6489; 1651–2251

Kerr AG (2005) Assessment of vertigo. Ann Acad Med Singapore 34(4):285–288, 0304–4602; 0304–4602

Leveque M, Siedermann L, Tran H, Language T, Ulmer E, Chays A (2010) Vestibular functions outcomes after vestibular neurectomy in Meniere's disease: can vestibular neurectomy provide complete vestibular differentiation? Auris Nasus Larynx 37(3):308–313, 0385–8146; 1879–1476

Palomar-Asenjo V, Boleas-Aguirre MS, Sanchez-Ferrandiz N, Perez Fernandez N (2006) Caloric and rotatory chair test results in patients with Meniere's disease. Otology and Neurotology, 27(7):945–50, 1531–7129

Prepageran N, Kisilevsky V, Tomlinson D, Ranalli P, Rutka J (2005) Symptomatic high frequency/acceleration vestibular loss: consideration of a new clinical syndrome of vestibular dysfunction. Acta Otolaryngol 125(1):48–54, 0001–6489; 0001–6489

Ruckenstein MJ et al (2002) Immunological and serological testing in patients with Meniere's disease. Otol Neurotol 23:517–521

Schonfeld U, Helling K, Clarke AH (2010) Evidence of unilateral isolated utricular hypofunction. Acta Otolaryngol 130(6):702–707, 0001–6489; 1651–2251

Seemungal BM (2007) Neurootological emergencies. Curr Opin Neurol 20(1):32–39, 1350–7540:1080–8248

Shojaku H, Watanabe Y, Yagi T, Takahashi M, Takeda T, Ikezono T, Ito J, Kubo T, Suzuki M, Takumida M, Takeda N, Furuya N, Yamashita H (2009) Changes in the characteristics of definite Meniere's disease over time in Japan: a long-term survey by the Peripheral Vestibular Disorder Research Committee of Japan, formerly the Meniere's Disease Research Committee of Japan. Acta Otolaryngol 129(2):155–160, 0001–6489; 1651–2553 (20)

Silverstein H, Smouha E, Jones R (1989) Natural history vs. surgery for Meniere's disease. Otolaryngol Head Neck Surg 100(1):6–16

Timmer FC, Zhou G, Guinan JJ, Kujawa SG, Hermann BS, Rauch SD (2006) VEMP in patients with Meniere's disease with drop attacks. Laryngoscope 116(5):776–779, 0023–852X

Ulubil SA, Eshraghi AA, Telischi FF, Angeli SI, Balkany TJ, Joy JJ (2008) Caloric function after endolymphatic sac surgery. Laryngoscope 118(2):295–299, 0023–852X; 0023–852X

Yardley L, Kirby S (2008) Understanding psychological distress in Ménière's disease. A systemic review. Psychol Health Med 13(3):257–273

Benign Paroxysmal Positional Vertigo (BPPV)

4

One of the commonest clinical conditions causing vertigo is the BPPV. It is seen in all age groups, but mainly the ageing population, though not necessarily so, as some younger patients with or without a history of head trauma may also present with it. About 0.6 % of the population is said to suffer with BPPV (Neuhauseur and Lampert 2009). This figure may vary in other parts of the world due to biological reasons.

In BPPV, vertigo is either initiated or propagated by the movement of head or by a body motion. Getting out of bed first thing in the morning may sometimes trigger off imbalance, just as an attempt to pick up an object from the floor or the top shelf might. In other words, any sudden movement of head may initiate a bout of vertigo. Each attack may last only a brief moment or may linger on for awhile. It is however never prolonged sensation of imbalance. The moment the patient acquires a stable position of the body and the head, the vertigo disappears. Such patients learn to live with the symptoms and are best advised to keep the body and head in alignment when getting out of the bed. They are also advised to avoid sudden postural changes, climbing the stairs without holding on the banister, picking an object from the floor or the shelf, etc.

Some of these patients have long-term symptoms of vertigo; others have only short and brief episodes. Many have a history of cervical osteoarthritis or spondylosis; others may develop it after a fall or head injury, a whiplash injury or a car accident.

The underlying pathology is considered to be a fault in the otolith bodies, which tend to gravitate to the bottom of the ampulla as expected on the movement of head, but failing to rise up back to the surface as normally they should, thus sending wrong signals to the delicate vestibulo-spinal tract system. Sometimes these calcified particles may indeed become detached and drift away into the semicircular canals. Until a few years ago, the management of the BPPV was mostly medicinal, but thanks to Mr. Epley, the task of helping out these patients has become simple, efficient and extremely rewarding.

A particularly frightening symptom, indeed a sign, is the appearance of a sudden fall. It typically happens without any prodromal symptoms, an aura or a warning.

S.H. Zaidi, A. Sinha, *Vertigo*,
DOI 10.1007/978-3-642-36485-3_4, © Springer-Verlag Berlin Heidelberg 2013

It is called the 'Tumarkin phenomenon'. It is also described as the 'otolith crisis of Tumarkin'.

Tumarkin described this condition in 1936 (Tumarkin 1936), attributing it to spontaneous mechanical deformation of the otolith organs, i.e. utricle and saccule, resulting in a rapid, sudden and alarming activation of the vestibular reflexes. These drop attacks may require repositioning of the otolith particles.

History and simple tests like Dix–Hallpike manoeuvre are nearly always diagnostic, though sometimes detailed vestibular investigations may be required. In order to understand the inner ear function in conditions such as Meniere's, vestibular neuritis or BPPV, which can all cause vertigo or imbalance, Wada et al. (2009) carried out a study of various modalities employed in the diagnosis of BPPV. They investigated their patients through PTA, calorimetry, etc. They observed higher rate of canal paresis on the affected side showing p values of <0.01. They also observed that the term of recovery at the first treatment was longer in a patient with canal paresis compared to those without. Their study also highlighted that fact that the horizontal semicircular canal and cochlea are important potential sits of lesions in posterior canal type of BPPV, and the posterior circular canal and otolith are already considered to be the sites of lesions.

Recently, evoked myogenic potentials have been employed as a useful tool in the diagnosis of BPPV. Many studies have shown that irrespective of the involvement of semicircular canals, the vestibular-evoked myogenic potentials have been found to have increased latencies (Mudduwa et al. 2010).

The diagnosis may pose a challenge in some acute situations as was noted by Zapala and colleagues (2006). They described a case of an acutely vertiginous patient who presented to the emergency department with simultaneous acute left labyrinthitis and left posterior canal benign paroxysmal positional vertigo (BPPV). Gaze nystagmus from the labyrinthitis hampered the diagnosis of the BPPV. However, once the BPPV was identified and treated, the patient's subjective vertigo improved rapidly. Such a mixed picture can indeed be quite confusing. Unless the clinician is aware of the possibility of a dual pathology as a cause of the symptoms, wrong management may ensue. It is therefore worth remembering that concomitant BPPV should not be overlooked when a diagnosis of acute labyrinthitis is made in the emergency department or on subsequent evaluation in the ENT department.

Considerable research goes on currently, on the subject of aetiopathogenesis as well as the biomechanics of BPPV. Rajgru and colleagues (2005) studied the biomechanics of horizontal canal BPPV. They believe that BPPV is the outcome of basophilic particles depositing in the semicircular canals. It involves the horizontal canal as a vestibular disorder characterised by bouts of horizontal ocular nystagmus induced during reorientation of the head relative to gravity. BPPV, according to this group, develops more frequently in the posterior canal. A history and a diagnostic test during which the head is rapidly pitched back in the plane of the posterior canal to provoke nystagmus can be extremely helpful. They explained that the horizontal canal variant is characterised by acute vertigo induced during such activities as rolling over in bed. They addressed the application of a morphologically descriptive 3-canal biomechanical model of the human membranous labyrinth to study gravity-dependent semicircular canal responses during this condition. The model estimated dynamic cupular and endolymph displacements elicited during HC-BPPV provocative diagnostic manoeuvres and canalith repositioning procedures (CRPs). The activation latencies in response to an HC-BPPV provocative diagnostic *test* were predicted to vary, depending upon the initial location of the canalith debris (e.g. within the HC lumen vs. in the ampulla). Obviously, it was a very sophisticated and research-oriented methodology, which may not be possible to be repeated in a busy clinic setting. Nevertheless, it was a highly scientific study.

They were confident that the results would explain why the onset latency of ocular nystagmus evoked by the Dix–Hallpike provocative manoeuvre for posterior canal BPPV are typically longer than the latencies evoked by analogous tests for HC-BPPV.

The model was further applied to assess the efficacy of 360° rotation CRP for the treatment of canalithiasis HC-BPPV. So far, this experimental work has only highlighted what could happen under controlled laboratory conditions. Obviously, further research is expected by these authors to publish in due course of time.

As we know, one of the presenting features of BPPV is its mode of onset of dizziness, which is often initiated, promoted or aggravated with the movement of head or changing the bodily posture in relation to head. This study helps identify the location of particle deposits in the canals, thus making the manoeuvring of the deposits more specific. In brief, if the patient complains of dizziness on turning in bed, it is most likely due to the deposits in the horizontal canal. If, however he feels giddy on extension of the head, in the plane of the posterior canals, he is likely to have the particles in the posterior canal.

Currently, Epley's manoeuvre remains the best form of treatment for BPPV. It provides dramatic and almost instantaneous relief. Recurrence of the symptoms may be relieved with the repetition of the manoeuvre.

4.1 Epley's Manoeuvre: How I Do It

The patient is explained the procedure and requested to sit upright on a couch. The patient is made to lie down in a supine position with the head rotated to the side causing the symptoms. The patient is instructed to remain in this position for about 5 min, encouraging the otoconia to gradually drift back towards the ampulla.

Next, the patient is instructed to turn the head 90° in the opposite direction and remain in that position for 5 min. The patient is then asked to roll over to the direction he is facing at the moment, retaining the head with nose down position for about 5 min. Finally, the patient is instructed to sit back and remain so for about 30 s. The procedure may have to be repeated up to 3 min.

This manoeuvre may be carried out by the patient himself at home. He is informed that at every step of the manoeuvre, he may feel momentarily dizzy (Epley 1980).

Epley's manoeuvre was the subject of a study conducted by Kaplan et al. (2005). The patients were treated with Epley's manoeuvre on the side that was more symptomatic and that had a greater velocity and amplitude of torsional nystagmus.

The patients were retreated according to symptoms and findings on follow-up visits: They describe their fruitful experience in treating most patients diagnosed with bilateral BPPV and treated with Epley's manoeuvre. All patients recovered after performing Epley's manoeuvre couple of times during a 3-month period. It was concluded that BiBPPV has typical characteristics and can be managed successfully with Epley's manoeuvre, though it may require a repeat effort.

Moon et al. (2005) agreed that BPPV is indeed provoked by head movements. They took a large sample of cohorts and retrospectively analysed clinical features of 1,692 patients. Their study discovered that majority (60.9 %) of patients had involvement of the posterior semicircular canals, while 31.9 % had horizontal canal, anterior canal in 2.2 and 5 % of them had mixed canals. They noted that about 87 % of patients were successfully treated with canalith repositioning through Epley's manoeuvre.

Leong and Golding-Wood (2008) showed the importance of care and caution in particle repositioning in BPPV. They agree with the general observation that particle repositioning procedures give consistent results for the treatment of benign positional paroxysmal vertigo (BPPV). However, they feel that little consideration has been given to the possibilities of bilateral disease. They therefore hypothesised that contralateral symptoms and signs suggestive of revealed or incipient BPPV as a complication of Epley's manoeuvre are a possibility. They carried out a study on prospective cohort of 198 cases over a period of 11 years. It was observed that 5 % of them developed contralateral symptoms and signs suggestive of revealed or incipient posterior canal BPPV within a fortnight of treatment.

They claimed that their novel observation has not been previously described. They also felt that it may influence the strategy for future management of patients with BPPV. Particle repositioning manoeuvres for the previously asymptomatic contralateral ear may need to be considered in a subset of patients with posterior canal BPPV who suffer contralateral symptoms after undergoing treatment for the original ear.

This paper duly challenged the routine practice of performing Epley's manoeuvre without much consideration about the contralateral ear. It certainly provides food for thought!

Effectiveness of canalith repositioning manoeuvre, in patients with BPPV, was investigated by Tevzadze and Shakarishvili (2007), in more than 200 patients. They found the BPPV affecting up to 21 % of vertiginous patients, characterised by episodes of vertigo associated with rapid changes in head position. All these patients who had a typical history of BPPV underwent neurological examination and the Dix–Hallpike manoeuvre with a view to detect posterior and anterior canal BPPV. Furthermore, a roll test was carried out to detect horizontal canal BPPV. The patients are then treated with Epley's repositioning. This study duly supplements the observation that timely and expertly applied Epley's manoeuvre certainly gives satisfactory relief to the patient suffering from BPPV.

It goes without saying that clinicians want to localise the fault in the semicircular canals in BPPV. One basic indicator is the history. If a patient feels dizzy on turning in bed, he may have a lesion in the horizontal canal. On the other hand, if one feels dizzy on head movement in the direction of the posterior canal, the deposits must be sitting in that canal. Clinical tests like the Dix–Hallpike tests will also give a clear indication. Part of the research carried out by Tevzadze and colleagues concentrated on this very aspect and established that it is possible to localise the site of otolith damage precisely in the labyrinthine maze and to look at the frequency of canal involvement.

After an exhaustive study, they found out that the posterior semicircular canal was involved in 170 patients. They also noted that 31 patients suffered from involvement of horizontal and 3 patients had problem with the anterior semicircular canal. They claim that after a single treatment session, the symptoms disappeared completely in 139 patients. Forty patients improved after 2 sessions, 16 patients after 3 sessions and 9 patients required multiple sittings. It goes without saying that practice makes on perfect. The experienced clinician or a scientist may yield better results in these manoeuvres than the one who may employ it on a few occasions only.

Generally speaking, one takes it for granted that BPPV is bilateral, but not necessarily so. Unilateral BPPV is difficult to establish, though it may cause the vertiginous symptoms. The current treatment remains the application of Epley's manoeuvre. In a recent study, Childs (2010) described that patients with unilateral vestibular hypofunction can be treated with adaptation, substitution and/or habituation exercises. Child also points out that patients with motion sensitivity can demonstrate improved tolerance to motion after performing habituation exercises.

Surgical management of BPPV is controversial and seldom if at all practiced. Seo et al. (2009) described the results of audiometry, calorimetry and VEMP in five patients who underwent surgical treatment described as 'plugging' of the posterior semicircular canal in chronic intractable BPPV. They claim that positional vertigo was resolved in all without affecting the hearing to more than 10 dB. Furthermore, they described that the VEMP did not vary more than 10 % from pre-surgical levels.

Of course, validity of such studies remains open to debate, as the data is so inadequate and the practice so limited that one may not have sufficient material to estimate the specificity and sensitivity of such a practice. We are quite happy with the conservative management of BPPV and see no reason to perform any surgical intervention in this benign and easily manageable condition.

For academic interest only such piece of information is useful for a clinician. Therefore, one more study is included here which demonstrates another facet of surgical management of BPPV, with possible loss of hearing.

Pournaras et al. (2008) claimed that the 'singular neurectomy' as described by Gacek in 1974 was an efficient procedure to control symptoms in a case of intractable benign paroxysmal positional vertigo (BPPV), with an acceptable risk of postoperative sensorineural hearing loss (SNHL). However, they postulated that this complication may not be a direct consequence of the surgical procedure but rather may be consecutive to the reactivation of the biological phenomenon that caused the BPPV. The authors also observed in one patient that BPPV may exist, although no nystagmus can be elicited by provocative manoeuvres.

Their results were quite optimistic. The authors reported that all patients were free of vertigo and considered their quality of life improved. The Hallpike's manoeuvre was negative in all cases. SNHL occurred in two patients, immediately after surgery in one and several months later in the second. The patient with a negative Hallpike's manoeuvre before surgery went back to work 3 weeks after surgery.

Such studies are worthy of note, albeit more confirmatory evidence for specificity and sensitivity would be required to supplement their observations. Besides, they have not gained popularity because non-invasive and simple procedures like the Epley's manoeuvre give more than satisfactory results. Therefore, surgical reports for BPPV are seldom and few and far between. One may add that the surgical application in such cases remains limited in application and confined to a few selected cases of chronic intractable BPPV. Obviously, it may be carried out in certain dedicated centres only. The fundamental rule of treatment is to provide relief to patient with less invasive procedures and preferably non-invasive methods if possible. The old days of large gashing wounds and heroic surgery are all but gone now. Currently, it is the era of minimally invasive key whole procedures. It may therefore be worthwhile to remember that surgical studies described above may have only an academic value in the modern-day management of BPPV. We are extremely satisfied with our results of Epley's manoeuvre, which takes only a few minutes, providing instant relief to the patient. One may repeat the procedure if necessary, in those who may have either less than satisfactory relief or failed to respond to the initial effort. We have no experience of surgical intervention in BPPV and find it quite difficult to recommend as a standard modality.

Some patients who require long-term management or a follow-up are referred to our vestibular lab, where our vestibular scientists repeat the manoeuvre if needed or, indeed, offer them more appropriate exercises.

4.2   Semont's Manoeuvre: How I Do It

This is another exercise that is often employed in the rehabilitative management of BPPV. Compared with the Epley's manoeuvre, it is relatively uncommon.

Its steps are as follows:

The patient is seated on an examination couch and the procedure explained. The head is then turned 45° horizontally towards the normal ear. The next step is to tilt the patient 105° so that the patient is lying on the affected side with the head supported. The patient is retained in this position for 3 min approximately. The next step is to swiftly bring the patient from sitting to lying position with the head supported and nose pointing towards the floor. This posture is retained for 3 min approximately. The patient is then moved back to a sitting position slowly to encourage the otoconia to return to their normal habitat in the utricle. As one can imagine, this manoeuvre is slightly cumbersome and remains a relatively uncommon way of managing BPPV.

The patient is advised to sleep in a semi-recumbent position for the next couple of nights after the Epley's or the Semont's manoeuvre. This position is best obtained by sleeping on a reclining chair with the head maintained at a 45° angle. He should also avoid all kinds of head bending, rotating and tilting movements for 2–3 days and avoid any movement of head that may provoke vertigo for about 1 week.

Then there are some other exercises like the Brandt-Daroff exercises that the vestibular team can advise if needed.

Sometimes, atypical cases of BPPV may be encountered. They are caused by movement of the otoconial bodies into the anterior/superior or lateral/horizontal canal. The reader is referred to standard textbooks for further study of these rare conditions.

And finally, here is a study that duly summarises the modes of treatment and validity in their application.

Exploring the treatments in complex vestibular conditions was the subject of an investigation by Childs (2010) who believed that those with unilateral vestibular hypofunction can be treated using adaptation, substitution and/or habituation exercises. Furthermore, patients with motion sensitivity can demonstrate improved tolerance to motion after performing habituation exercises. Patients with bilateral vestibular loss will benefit from substitution and adaptation exercises. Each patient requires a treatment regime that is individualised and appropriate to address their impairments. Often the treatment is determined through the evaluation process. The task that causes the patient's complaints, whether it is dizziness, imbalance and/or issues with eye–head coordination, often becomes the treatment of choice, gradually increasing difficulty as appropriate and safe. Patients with TBI who have concomitant vestibular dysfunction are a challenging population to treat. One has to be aware of cognitive deficits that may interfere with or prolong treatment as well as the many other neurological deficits that may be present because of the brain injury. For example, attempting to perform the canalith repositioning manoeuvre on a patient status post-TBI when they are not able to comprehend the reasoning behind the treatment can lead to agitation or behavioural issues. Communication with the patient's primary doctor is a necessity so that the team is always on the same page about the approach to the treatment.

And that is absolutely true. Keeping the family physician on board in the management of all vertiginous patients must be the fundamental rule. After all, there are numerous other causes of vertigo besides those discussed here which may fall outside the domain of an otolaryngologist, and the family doctor would know best how to cope with them. Timely referral of a vertiginous patient to the relevant speciality should be a rule rather than an exception. This particularly applies to cardiac and diabetic patients, who may often have multiple causes of their dizziness, each needing due attention.

Case Report

P born in 1946 was referred to our vestibular lab and was seen in March 2010. He described movement-provoked dizziness since last 6 months. He also noticed momentary loss of balance on getting out of bed and on looking up to the ceiling or down onto the floor, lasting a few seconds only. He also noticed dizziness on turning his head to the right. Mr. P also reported true rotatory vertigo on lying down in bed.

Recently, he also had a week long rotatory vertigo, accompanied by nausea but no vomiting. During the attack, he was able to walk around but felt worse when making sudden head movements. His GP prescribed him a short course of betahistine, which helped him, but his motion-provoked imbalance continued as such.

P had no problem with hearing. For the past week or so, he had noticed momentary spells of 'dulled hearing' with tinnitus. He did not notice any changes in hearing or tinnitus coinciding with dizzy spells. He said that his ear felt blocked more on the left than on the right side. He suffered from headaches lasting a day or two. He also had cervical osteoarthritis and wondered if his headaches could stem from. He had pains and aches in the neck and felt 'grinding' sensation in his neck on turning his head. He also complained of numbness of the right side of his face lasting couple of days, but it did not coincide with dizziness. His facial nerve was normal on each side. He took several medications for his acidity, hypercholesterolemia, etc.

The otoscopy was normal, as was the tympanometry. Ipsilateral acoustic reflexes were present at stimulus levels within normal range, bilaterally using a 1 kHz stimulus. PTA revealed a mild high-frequency sensorineural loss bilaterally.

On functional testing, Mr. P was able to maintain his balance with reduced visual and proprioceptive inputs. Ocular motor testing using VNG revealed no spontaneous, gaze-evoked neck positional or rebound nystagmus. No abnormalities were detected upon testing of random saccades and smooth pursuit. Neck positional testing revealed no nystagmus or subjective sensation. Monothermal warm water caloric testing revealed approximately equal and robust responses. Visual fixation index was normal. Dix–Hallpike test revealed no nystagmus or subjective responses on the right; on the left side, nystagmus was observed, and a modified Epley's manoeuvre was performed on this side initially. Mr. P also experienced subjective sensation. Upon further examination of the recording, the nystagmus was found to be right-beating horizontal (ageotropic) with a 2 s onset and 9 s duration. This was highly suggestive of a BPPV of the right horizontal canal so a log roll to the left with fast head movements was performed. Mr. P felt relieved.

Mr. P was informed that he may have to return for reaped manoeuvre if the symptoms reoccurred. Mr. P was also referred by his GP for the physiotherapy of his neck.

Case Report

P, 70 years of age, was seen in our vestibular lab in May 2010. She gave a history of rotatory vertigo provoked by getting out of bed briskly on sudden postural changes. Also, she felt dizzy on looking up or down. She also veered to the right on walking. She has previously taken SERC with some benefit.

Mrs. P had noted a slight fall in her hearing in the recent months, particularly on the left side. She wore a digital aid in her left ear. Her tinnitus in left ear caused her much distress as she noticed it to worsen in the last 2 months.

She also had cervical spondylosis, backaches and hypertension for which she was consulting her GP.

Dix–Hallpike testing did not produce a nystagmus or initiate any subjective sensation of vertigo on the left side. On the right side, a right-beating tensional nystagmus was seen lasting about 11 s, after a 2 s delay. A modified Epley's manoeuvre was performed on the right with symptomatic relief.

He was given a follow-up telephonic appointment to check if he required any further manoeuvre. She was also referred for tinnitus counselling.

References

Childs LA (2010) Assessing vestibular dysfunction. Exploring treatments of a complex condition. Rehab Manag 23(6):24–50, 0899–623

Epley JM (1980) New dimensions of benign paroxysmal positional vertigo. Otolaryngol Head Neck Surg 88(5):599–605, PMID 7443266

Kaplan DM, Nash M, Niv A, Kraus M (2005) Management of bilateral benign paroxysmal positional vertigo. Otolaryngol Head Neck Surg 133(5):769–773, 0194–5998

Leong AC, Golding-Wood D (2008) Contralateral incipient posterior canal benign positional paroxysmal vertigo: complication after Epley's manoeuvre. Laryngoscope 118(11):2087–2090, 0023–852X; 1531–4995

Moon SY, Kim BK, Kim JI, Lee H, Son SI, Kim KS, Rhee CK, Han GC, Lee WS (2005) Clinical characteristics of BPPV in Korea. A study. J Korean Med Sci 21:539–543

Mudduwa R, Kara N, Whelan D, Banerjee A (2010) Vestibular evoked myogenic potentials: review. J Laryngol Otol 124:1043–1050

Neuhauseur HK, Lampert T (2009) Vertigo: epidemiologic aspects. Semin Neurol 29(5):473–481. doi:10.1055/s-0029-1241043. PMID 19834858

Pournaras I, Kos I, Guyot JP (2008) Benign paroxysmal positional vertigo: a series of eight singular neurectomies. Acta Otolaryngol 128(1):5–8

Rajgru SM, Ifediba MA, Rabitt RD (2005) Biomechanics of horizontal canal benign positional vertigo. J Vestib Res 15(4):203–214, 0957–4271

Seo T, Hashimoto M, Saka N, Sakagami M (2009) Hearing and vestibular functions after plugging surgery for the posterior semicircular canal. Acta Otolaryngol 129(11):1148–1152, 0001–6489; 1651–2251

Tevzadze N, Shakarishvili R (2007) Effectiveness of canalith repositioning manoeuvers (CRM) in patients with benign paroxysmal positional vertigo (BPPV). Georgian Med News 148–149:40–44, 1512–0112

Tumarkin A (1936) The otolithic catastrophe. Br Med J 2:175

Wada S, Naganuma H, Tokumasu K, Oakamoto M (2009) Inner ear function tests in cases of posterior canal-type BPPV. Int Tinnitus J 15(1):91–93, 0946–5448

Zapala DA, Shapiro SA, Lundy LB, Leming DT (2006) Simultaneous acute superior nerve neurolabyrinthitis and benign paroxysmal positional vertigo. J Am Acad Audiol 17(7): 481–486; quiz 531–532, 1050–0545

Vestibular Migraine

5

Headache is usually a symptom of an underlying cause. Hypertension, for instance, is a known cause of headaches. It may be a benign headache without any underlying pathology, as many headaches are, but sometimes, it may be so intense as to lead to photophobia, phonophobia and dizziness.

Migraine is an extremely unpleasant form of headache, which may attack the customer in the form of a solitary crippling and debilitating attack or in clusters. Beside excruciating headache, photophobia, nausea and sickness, it may also cause dizziness.

Basilar migraine is a known cause of vertigo. Most clinicians are fully aware of this condition and deal with it on a regular basis. Vestibular migraine is clearly a different clinical entity.

For an unknown reason, vestibular migraine is still waiting to be recognised as a common cause of vertigo. We believe that it is much commoner than many other well-known causes.

Contemporary International Classification of Headaches Disorders does not recognise vertigo as a migrainous symptom. The ICHD wants to see at least two posterior circulation manifestations lasting between 5 and 60 min followed by a migraine headache (Lempert and Neuhauseur 2009). As a matter of fact, vestibular migraine is the second most frequent cause of recurrent vertigo with a lifetime history of recurring episodes (Neuhauser and Lampert 2009). It does not always accompany an attack of intense headache so typically experienced by migrainous patients; however, it is quite a well-known phenomenon that a patient with repeated bouts of migraine may develop vestibular symptoms. A full-fledged case of migraine begins with an aura and is nearly always accompanied with nausea, vomiting, photophobia, phonophobia and unbearable headache. Sometimes half-sided headache is confused with fulminating sinusitis, which can be excluded by simple clinical examination of the nose with a nasoendoscope.

Cluster headache is also a common condition which may sometimes precipitate vertigo. Typically the cluster headaches affect the weak and the psychologically vulnerable, usually young people. It comes in bouts with intermission in between

S.H. Zaidi, A. Sinha, *Vertigo*,
DOI 10.1007/978-3-642-36485-3_5, © Springer-Verlag Berlin Heidelberg 2013

the attacks. There are some people with rather volatile personalities, in whom a cluster headache may also be accompanied with sensation of rotation of objects.

Many young women develop migraine or migraine-like symptoms just a day or two before their menstruation. It has often been described as premenstrual tension headache. The exact cause remains unknown, but it is an established entity often seen in clinical practice. Sometimes, the intensity and duration may be related to the intensity of menstruation, as menorrhagia may be associated with prolonged duration of migrainous headaches.

What causes migraine or the cluster headaches is discussed at length in major textbooks. Suffice it to say that we do not know the cause for certain. It is presumed that it is related to an adverse response of the autonomic nervous system resulting in rapid and spontaneous release of histamine, bradykinin, serotonin and a multitude of hitherto unidentified chemical mediators. It results in vasodilatation of the capillaries in rather narrow spaces of the skull, causing the symptoms of migraine.

It is also seen that these patients do respond adversely to certain diets such as bananas, some chocolates, red grapes or red wine, a Chinese salt called Ajinomoto and some forms of cheese.

Some people are susceptible to many food elements and additives and react adversely to substances like tyramine, phenylalanine, phenolic flavonoids, alcohol, sodium nitrate and monosodium glutamate. The reactive response is sometimes also called the Chinese syndrome.

Clinically, the vestibular migraine presents with attacks of spontaneous or slow and steady vertigo lasting from a few seconds to days. Migrainous accompaniments such as headache, phonophobia, photophobia or auras are common but not mandatory. Cochlear symptoms may be associated but are mostly mild and nonprogressive. During acute attacks, one may find central spontaneous or positional nystagmus and, less commonly, unilateral vestibular hypofunction. In the symptom-free interval, vestibular testing adds little to the diagnosis as findings are mostly minor and non-specific. In the absence of controlled studies, treatment of VM is adopted from the migraine sphere comprising avoidance of triggers, stress management as well as pharmacotherapy for acute attacks and prophylaxis.

It was noted in a study that in migraine polyneuropathy in 32 % compared with 18 % in BV patients without cerebellar signs. Hypoacusis occurred bilaterally in 25 % and unilaterally in 6 % of all patients (Lempert and Neuhauseur 2009; Neuhauser and Lampert 2009; Neuhauseur et al. 2001).

Neuhauser and Brevern had investigated the epidemiology of vestibular migraine. In this paper, claiming the lifetime prevalence of migraine to be about 14 % and dizziness/vertigo affecting 20–30 % of the population. They believe that the vestibular migraine affects 1 % of the general population.

Neuhauser criteria for migrainous vertigo is accepted by most clinicians as gold standard for evaluating this clinical condition (Neuhauseur et al. 2001). It defines the parameters under the categories of Definite and Probable. The definite symptoms include:

1. Episodic vestibular symptoms of moderate severity.
2. Migraine according to International Headache Society criteria.

3. One or more of the features during at least two vertiginous attacks: migrainous headache, headache, photophobia, photophobia, an aura.
4. Other diagnoses excluded by appropriate tests.
Amongst the probable cases, they have included:
1. Episodic vestibular symptoms of moderate severity.
2. One or more of features, namely, migraine headaches, migraine symptoms during vertigo, migraine-specific triggers and response to anti-migraine therapy.
3. Other diagnoses excluded.

Many other workers such as Kahmke and Kaylie reviewed the epidemiology and association of migraine with vertigo recently, quoting many studies such as those conducted by (Radtke and Neausheur et al. 2011).

Interestingly enough, no consensus was reached on the definite figure amongst all these workers, making the issue more complex than it ought to be.

Tomanovic and Bergenius (2010) observed that migraine is often overshadowed with many other symptoms particularly dizziness, blurring of vision, photophobia and some vasovagal symptoms. They studied different types of dizziness in patients with peripheral vestibular diseases, their prevalence and relation to migraine. It was duly pointed out that beside spontaneous attacks of vertigo or unsteadiness, other features, i.e. drop attacks, illusions that the room or body is tilted, 'walking on pillows' or 'stepping into a hole', occur without precipitating head movement in almost 50 % of patients with peripheral vestibular dysfunctions. The sensation of static tilt was closely connected to migraine and Meniere's disease in their view. They recorded the prevalence of the different symptoms with respect to vestibular diagnosis and its relation to migraine by collecting data from 100 patients with Meniere's disease, benign paroxysmal positional vertigo (BPPV) or unilateral peripheral vestibular impairment (UPVI). The results were analysed with respect to vestibular diagnosis with migraine as a secondary diagnosis. They discovered that spontaneous attacks of vertigo or unsteadiness occurred in 74 and 48 % of patients, respectively. Vertigo was significantly more often reported in patients with Meniere's and BPPV. In patients with BPPV, the duration of spontaneous vertigo was shorter than in patients with Meniere's.

No doubt this study further highlights the dilemma presented by a dizzy patient. A clinician must be cognisant of the various colours of dizziness. Each patient must be assessed based upon individual history, thorough clinical examination and the diagnostic tests.

The possibility of a common pathophysiology between migraine and Meniere's cannot be ruled out. As a matter of fact, they both might be cousins in a manner of speaking. The overlap between migraine and vertigo has been the subject of a study by Sheppard (2006) and colleagues. They reviewed a significant body of literature demonstrating a relationship between migrainous disorders and dizziness. They agreed that in the characterisations of the migraine-associated dizziness, the signs and symptoms show overlap with Meniere's disease. Sufficient literature is available, beginning with Meniere himself, suggesting a relationship between Meniere's disease and migraine-associated dizziness. This implicates a possible underlying link in pathogenesis. This review article presented a discussion of the overlap in signs and symptoms between the two disorders. The author also suggested to differentiate between the disorders based on recent literature protocols and use of test results. He believes that vestibular and balance rehabilitation programs have a role in both of the disorders but differ in the overall management aspects of the disorders.

In cases of migrainous vertigo, a history combined with normal caloric response may be sufficient evidence to treat the underlying cause, i.e. migraine, rather than prescribe betahistines, which is a fairly common practice.

Just like many vertiginous conditions, the fact is that migraine does require a comprehensive history taking and a thorough clinical examination. Celebisoy et al. (2008) looked at the clinical features of migrainous vertigo in some detail.

They pointed out that migrainous vertigo (MV) is accepted as a common cause of episodic vertigo. They agree with the general opinion that peripheral or central vestibular localisation of the deficit in this condition as well as the pathophysiology is unclear. This prospective study was designed to assess the clinical features of vestibular migraine and to search for the localisation of the vestibular pathology. The study involved comparison of 35 patients of migrainous vertigo, 20 patients with migraine alone and 20 healthy cohorts as controls.

They performed detailed neurological and ontological tests, between the attacks. None of the controls or the patients with migraine alone showed ocular motor deficits or caloric test abnormalities. They also noted that three patients in the migrainous vertigo group showed saccadic pursuit (8.6 %), one of them showing saccadic hypometria.

Caloric test results revealed unilateral caloric hypofunction in seven patients. Their findings during the symptom-free period revealed that peripheral vestibular dysfunction was more common than a central pathology.

It is evident from this study that migrainous vertigo indeed demands a careful evaluation of the patient and can be easily diagnosed with some basic tests routinely employed in most vestibular lab, as is our practice also. A few case reports from our clinical setup are described here to supplement the statement.

One has to admit that observing specifically for nystagmus in case of migraine is not a common clinical practice; however, when the patient presents with vertigo, it is mandatory to look for nystagmus. We have seldom found positive evidence of horizontal nystagmus in cases who presented to us in the outpatient in a phase when they still had migraine, though subacute or residual in nature, for evaluation of a vestibular cause of vertigo. In a study Polensek and Tusa (2010) gave due importance to the clinical sign of nystagmus in migrainous vertigo. They believe that an estimated one-fourth to one-third of patients with migraine will experience vertigo associated with their migraine.

In this study, they looked at the features that characterise eye movements of patients presenting with nystagmus during attacks of migrainous vertigo.

It was a retrospective study of 26 patients presenting with nystagmus during an acute vestibular migraine. All patients were examined while symptomatic during a migraine spell and also while asymptomatic. All patients underwent tests of vestibular function with either a traditional calorimetry or an electronystagmography.

As mentioned above, in our experience, we have not found nystagmus as a common observation in vestibular migraine. It could well be due to the simple reason that we usually see a patient during a quiescent phase, when the symptoms have already settled down. ENT clinicians would seldom, if at all, see an acute case of migraine; as often enough, it is such a debilitating experience that the victim of this unruly headache feels best to tide it over with simple but effective measures learnt through the past experience, rather than wait in the consulting room of an ENT specialist for a length of time. In an acute situation, the family physician or an urgent care clinician must, however, look for a nystagmic beat in a volatile attack of vestibular migraine. With patience and a keen eye for minute details, he may be duly rewarded.

The study demonstrated that the most common patient was a female of premenopausal age. Spontaneous nystagmus was seen in 19 % of patients, and nystagmus provoked by horizontal head shaking was seen in 35 %. Nystagmus could be provoked with positional testing in 100 % of symptomatic patients with fixation blocked.

The positional nystagmus most commonly was sustained, of low velocity, and could be horizontal, vertical or torsional. Conventional calorimetry or rotational chair tests obtained during symptom-free intervals were normal in all patients.

It was therefore concluded by these authors that although characteristics of the nystagmus are quite variable during vestibular migraine, the finding on examination of low-velocity, sustained nystagmus with positional testing in a young to middle-aged adult patient presenting with vertigo, nausea and headache is highly suggestive of vestibular migraine as long as the nystagmus dissipates when the patient is free of symptoms.

This study is highly profitable for a clinician, as nystagmus is the only objective feature of vertigo, which as we have discussed *ad nauseum* is a subjective feeling. The only flaw with this study is that it could well be an atypical case of vestibular migraine with nystagmus. Obviously, we would like to investigate this further in our patients as surely others with similar interests may do too.

Nystagmus has been discussed at some length in this book and is certainly the most important observable sign of vertigo.

Most patients with migraine develop their own strategies for combating their grief. One common remedy practised by many is to take a day off and go to bed. They may or may not be able to sleep, but with the help of basic analgesics, most would get some relief after a day's rest, usually in a quiet, darkened room without any distractions such as the TV or music.

Many specific anti-migrainous medicines are also available and often quite helpful. But the fundamental advice to these patients is to identify the trigger factors and avoid them. Fortunately, the frequency and the intensity of migraine decline with age.

The management of migrainous vertigo is basically medicinal. It is however claimed that rehabilitation therapy has positive contributory role to play in this rather troublesome clinical condition.

Wrisley et al. (2002) investigated the efficacy of physical therapy for patients with vestibular disorders with and without a history of migraine. They investigated 30 patients with both a history of migraine and a diagnosis of vestibulopathy considered unrelated to migraine by a retrospective chart review. These patients completed the Dizziness Handicap Inventory, the Activities-Specific Balance Confidence Scale, the Dynamic Gait Index, and the Timed up and Go Test and rated the severity of their dizziness on an analogue scale of 0–100.

It should be noted though that such tests, however, are not routinely performed in an average vestibular lab and are mentioned here as a part of a study carried out elsewhere.

Their results showed significant differences within both groups between initial evaluation and discharge in each of the assessment measures used. Patients with a history of migraine demonstrated worse scores on all outcome measures than did the patients without a history of migraine. There were no statistically significant differences between the two groups' scores before and after therapy except for the total Dizziness Handicap Inventory score at discharge ($p < 0.05$). The authors concluded from this study that patients with vestibular disorders with or without a history of migraine demonstrated improvements in both subjective and objective measures of balance after physical therapy. Those with a history of migraine perceived a greater handicap from dizziness than did patients without a history of migraine that was greater than the difference in physical function performance measures between groups.

Furman et al. (2003) looked at the vestibular migraine as an essential contributor to chronic vertiginous diseases. They noted that the vestibular symptoms occur frequently in patients with migraine. They reviewed the diagnostic criteria for migraine-related vestibular symptoms and proposed to develop a pathophysiological model for the interface between migraine and the vestibular system.

These workers believe that the epidemiological link between migraine and vestibular symptoms and signs suggests shared pathogenetic mechanisms. They highlighted the links between the vestibular nuclei, the trigeminal system and thalamocortical processing centres which provide the basis for the development of a pathophysiological model of migraine-related vertigo. In this paper, they mentioned that during the last year, several studies had increased understanding of the relationship between migraine and vestibular symptoms. In their work, they found that motion sickness and allodynia in migrainous patients supported the importance of central mechanisms of sensitisation for migraine-related vestibular symptoms. Another study by the same author earlier on had demonstrated effective treatment of vertigo with migraine therapy. The identification of migrainous vertigo, however, in their view is hampered by a lack of standardised assessment criteria for both clinical and research practices.

Furman et al. believe that an understanding of the relationship between migraine and the vestibular system increases knowledge of the pathogenesis of both migraine and vertigo. In addition, they mentioned that several studies have identified successful treatment, with standard migraine therapies, of vestibular symptoms in patients with both migraine and vertigo. In their view the use of a standardised tool for assessment to identify this unique population of patients will help future studies to test both the pathological model and effective treatment. And that is exactly the point that we have made in our discussions and previous publications and sincerely propose in this clinical guide. It cannot be said without detailed and comprehensive epidemiological research; one may never be able to identify the exact extent of burden of disease that vestibular migraine poses to the human community at global level.

In the neuro-otological circles, vestibular migraine is accepted as a distant clinical entity. However, it remains a controversial diagnosis in certain neurological circles and is not recognised in the international falsification of headaches disorders (CHD 11), which recognises vertigo as one of non-aural symptoms of basilar type migraine.

Many excellent papers provide evidence from epidemiological studies duly supported by clinical findings, and the differential diagnoses with other causes like BPPV and Meniere's, that vestibular migraine is indeed a clinical entity worthy of due recognition. A denial of the reality may only amplify the magnitude of menace of vertigo in many populations. Further studies may be carried out through more specific tests like the biomarker's identification, genetic studies and field trials to confirm the fact.

Migraine is a chameleon. It may present in many different colours. Vasomotor instability may have a role to play in such patients, as some may be emotionally labile. Phobias may also lead to migrainous symptoms in some situations. One such patient had the fear of life whenever she went out and about, especially in the glass houses and tall buildings of the new shopping malls. She would develop intense headache with throbbing pain across the forehead, dizziness, nausea and sickness. She was known to tremble and sometime fall down only to be rushed to the A/E with no long-term treatment. In the ENT department, she was thoroughly investigated for a possible Meniere's with normal caloric responses and a normal VNG. Eventually, she was referred to a psychiatrist who discovered that her underlying problem was indeed of psychogenic nature. She was sexually abused as a child in a shopping mall and was living with that fear. Each time she saw the glass walls she would recall the tragedy and develop the symptoms described here.

Case Report
Mrs. P, aged 42 years, was referred to the vestibular lab for further investigations in January 2010. Her imbalance began approximately 4 years ago. Upon getting up from her bed, she experienced rotatory vertigo that persisted for roughly 2 days, though it bothered her about a fortnight. She ascribed it to a family bereavement. Over the next 2 years, she received medication periodically, until her symptoms disappeared. In August 2009, she experienced an awful episode of vertigo which was rotatory, with high-pitched tinnitus, and nausea lasting for about 2–3 weeks. Her symptoms were brought under control by betahistine, though she still felt unsteady,

describing her feeling as a gentle ride on a boat. Additionally, she experienced momentary dizziness upon rolling to her right side in the bed. Her otoscopy and PTA were normal. Tympanometry showed Eustachian dysfunction on the right side with normal function on the left. More importantly, she also suffered from headache simultaneous to her dizziness. She also said that she had migraines with seeing spots in her vision as if someone was 'shining a torch in her eyes', even with eyes closed. She also felt tingling sensation on her face.

She had no complaints about her hearing though occasionally echoic, which is relieved by popping the ears. She had whiplash injury a couple of years ago requiring physiotherapy and still felt aches and pains in her neck particularly on turning her head to the right.

Functional balance testing showed that she was able to maintain her balance with reduced proprioceptive and visual inputs. Using videonystagmography, oculomotor nerve testing revealed no spontaneous, rebound or gaze-evoked nystagmus and no abnormalities of smooth pursuit or saccades. A Dix–Hallpike manoeuvre also showed no nystagmus for either side, although she did report a subjective dizzy sensation when sitting up from the right-sided manoeuvre. Bithermal calorimetry revealed no significant canal paresis or directional preponderance.

It was therefore concluded that she did not have a peripheral or central lesion. Her most likely diagnosis could be migraine-induced vertigo, requiring medical treatment.

Case Report

P was 43 years of age, who presented with the complaints of true rotatory vertigo and was sent to our vestibular lab for further evaluation. She said that her vertigo was mostly noticed as she got out of bed but came and went throughout the day. The spells had worsened during the last 8–9 months since they first began. She denied any history of nausea but felt that she might pass out, though it did not actually happen. There were no provoking factors and she felt relieved with prochlorperazine.

She also reported suffering with repeated headaches mainly frontal, along with photophobia and phonophobia. The headaches did not alleviate with sleep. She was unsure as to what extent her headaches coincided with her vertigo, but she said that it appeared that the headaches were normally followed by vertigo. However, vertigo could occur without a headache. Additionally, she also described a yellow/red visual aura while she felt dizzy but could not recall if this happened during headaches. She also complained to pain below her right ear, which she thought could also be accompanied with a tingling sensation in her face. There was no history of tinnitus or hearing loss.

Upon otoscopy and local examination of the ear, nothing significant was found. Her facial nerve on either side was intact and normal, and the trigeminal nerve did not show any untoward features either. She was a bit sensitive to the otoscopy examination on the right side. Her most recent audiogram indicated normal levels bilaterally except at a loss of 25–30 dB at 6 and 8 kHz, bilaterally. Tympanometry was normal on either side.

Functional balance testing showed that the patient was able to maintain her balance with reduced proprioceptive and visual inputs. Using videonystagmography, oculomotor nerve testing revealed no spontaneous, rebound or gaze-evoked nystagmus and no abnormalities of smooth pursuit or random saccades. Bithermal water caloric testing revealed no significant canal paresis or directional preponderance. Her visual fixation index was normal.

In conclusion, the results showed no evidence of peripheral vestibular lesion or of a central lesion. It was therefore thought that her symptoms of headaches, visual auras, photophobias and phonophobia along with episodic vertiginous symptoms could be of migrainous origin.

Case Report

P born in 1969 was seen in our vestibular lab in January 2010. She found it difficult to describe some of her symptoms but said that her spells of dizziness began in August 2009. She described an initial episode of headache, dizziness, nausea and vomiting which hit her in the middle of the night. She apparently attempted to get out of bed but fell back down. She was bed ridden for 2 months and was on medication to control her symptoms. Since then, she has had several bouts of dizziness lasting about 5 min, particularly on looking up or down or turning to her right side. She also notices dizziness when sitting or lying down about three or four times a week. She found it difficult to describe her dizziness clearly but denied any rotatory vertigo. She also said that her headaches seemed to be more intense during her menstruation, finding it hard to walk straight and failing to control her weight on her right leg.

Mrs. P also complained of noticing her hearing to be worse with a background noise. She had a tapping tinnitus bilaterally, when lying in bed which she had noticed over the past 2 years. She noticed ear ache and daily episodes of headaches on the right side accompanied with photo- and phonophobia. She apparently saw 'heat waves' in her field of vision, particularly when she had intense headaches and dizziness. She described noticing a purple ball in her field of vision on her left side about 4 days ago. She had once hit her head on the floor and lost consciousness in May 2009.

The otoscopy was normal on both sides. PTA showed normal levels bilaterally, as did the tympanogram.

On functional testing Mrs. P was not able to maintain her balance with reduced visual inputs (vestibular and proprioceptive inputs present). VNG showed no spontaneous, gaze-evoked or rebound nystagmus. No abnormalities were detected upon testing of random saccades or smooth pursuit. Dix–Hallpike testing produced a subjective sensation bilaterally, although no nystagmus was noted; however, the patient did have difficulties in keeping her eyes open. Calorimetry was deferred temporarily and carried out a week later. Both Dix–Hallpike testing was negative bilaterally. Warm water calorimetry screening test revealed robust and equal responses bilaterally. Visual fixation index was also within normal limits on both sides.

The conclusion was made that Mrs. P did not have any peripheral or central vestibular problem, and the history was almost diagnostic of vestibular migraine.

Case Report

P was born in 1982 and was seen in our vestibular lab in April 2010. She *reported* spells of rotatory vertigo beginning a couple of months ago, provoked by standing up from a sitting position, getting out of bed, walking briskly, walking upstairs and lifting her head after bending forward. The spells lasted only a few minutes, but she thought she might fall down with the attack.

P gave a history of severe headaches beginning a few months prior to the onset of dizziness. The headache could hit her every couple of day lasting a few weeks. They could be unilateral or bilateral. They were associated with photophobia and visual aura. She also experienced nausea but had felt sick only once. She said specifically that the headaches and dizziness could happen simultaneously or independently.

P denied a hearing loss but had intermittent ticking tinnitus in both eras lasting only a few minutes. Tinnitus was not associated with the dizziness and could occur at the time of headaches also. She also mentioned of pressure sensation in both her ears with her headaches and had problems travelling by air.

She had a history of palpitation, but her ECG was reported to be normal. There was no history of angina *per se* nor any other heart disease. She, however, had thyrotoxicosis and took carbimazole on a daily basis.

Her otoscopy was normal, with normal middle ear pressure bilaterally on tympanometry. PTA revealed a 35 dB loss at 8 kHz on the left side.

On functional testing she was able to maintain her balance with reduced visual and proprioceptive inputs. Testing of random saccades and smooth pursuit using VNG revealed no abnormalities. Dix–Hallpike tests revealed no nystagmus, bilaterally, but some dizziness upon sitting on the left was experienced by P.

It was concluded that she did not have a peripheral or a central vestibular pathology or indeed a BPPV. The only other possibility was that she suffered from vestibular migraine.

Case Report

P born in 1958 was referred to our vestibular lab for diagnostic assessment. She was seen in Jan 2011 when she reported that for the past 12 months, she had been prone to stumbling and falling. Walking downstairs made her hold on to the banister, and she felt unsteady on walking up or down. She had a history of fall on a few occasions. The falls happened without a warning and did not result in any untoward end like unconsciousness or an injury. She denied any true vertigo associated with her fall. In the past she had felt unsteady, dizzy and unwell. She had sustained a road traffic accident 30 years ago.

Ms. P felt that her hearing had in fact deteriorated during the past 1 year. And felt that her left ear was worse of the two. She denied any fluctuation of hearing around the times of dizziness. She had bilateral intermittent tinnitus for the past few years. There was nothing of note on otoscopy. Her general health was poor as she had hypertension, hypercholesterolemia, obesity and headaches. She suffered with migraines with a history of photophobia and diplopia as well as some difficult in judging the distances. For instance, when reaching out to pick up an object, she would miss the object with her hand and overshoot it.

No abnormalities were detected on PTA except an island of hearing loss down to 25 dB at 2 and 4 kHz, marginally more on the left than right side.

Ocular motor nerve testing using VNG revealed no spontaneous nystagmus or a gaze-evoked nystagmus when fixation was present. Without fixation, a slight right-beating nystagmus was present in the centre, rightward and leftward gaze positions; however, this was below the level deemed clinically significant. Smooth pursuit eye movements had produced bilateral gain. Saccadic eye movements had latency and velocity within normal limits but borderline accuracy with some glissades particularly upon leftward eye movement. No rebound nystagmus was detected. Ms. P was able to maintain her balance with reduced visual and proprioceptive inputs. Because of an uncontrolled BP, calorimetry was not attempted. The head thrust was negative. The head shaking test revealed a consistent right-beating nystagmus of slightly greater amplitude than recorded during gazing testing. The clinical rotating chair test provoked nystagmus within normal limits bilaterally. In conclusion the abnormal saccadic and smooth pursuit eye movements were thought to be suggestive of a central vestibular problem. The nystagmus observed upon head shaking test could be suggestive of a peripheral vestibular lesion; however, right-beating nystagmus was also observed upon gaze testing without fixation. Therefore, it was not possible to conclude whether the nystagmus seen post-head shaking was the result of a peripheral lesion or it was spontaneous nystagmus. She was not a typical patient of vestibular lesion; hence, vestibular rehab was not suggested at this time.

Ms. P was already under the care of the neurologists for the treatment of her migraine with a history of falls. A request was sent for a review. The strong possibility was that she suffered from vestibular migraine.

References

Celebisoy N, Gokcay F, Sirin H, Bicak N (2008) Migrainous vertigo: clinical, oculographic and posturographic findings. Cephalalgia 28(1):72–77, 0333–1024; 1468–2982

Furman JM, Marcus DA, Balaban C (2003) Migrainous vertigo: development of a pathogenic model and structured diagnostic interview. Curr Opin Neurol 16(1):5–13

Lempert T, Neuhauser HK (2009) Epidemiology of vertigo, migraine, and vestibular migraine. J Neurol 256:333–338

Neuhauser HK, Lampert T (2009) Vertigo epidemiologic aspects. Semin Neurol 29(5):473–481. doi:10.1055/s-0029-1241043. PMID19834858

Neuhauser HK, Leopoldo M, von Breven M et al (2001) The interrelations of migraine, vertigo and migrainous vertigo. Neurology 56:436–441

Polensek SH, Tusa RJ (2010) Nystagmus during attacks of vestibular migraine: an aid in diagnosis. Audiol Neurootol 15(4):241–260, 1420–3030, 1421–9700

Radtke A, Neuhauser HK, von Brevenern M (2011) Vetibular migraine. Cephalalgia 31:901–913

Sheppard NT (2006) Differentiation of Meniere's disease and migraine-associated dizziness: a review. J Am Acad Audiol 17(1):69–80, 1050–0545

Tomanovic T, Bergenius J (2010) Different types of dizziness in patients with peripheral vestibular diseases – their prevalence and relation to migraine. Acta Otolaryngol 130(9):1024–1030, 0001–6489; 1651–2251

Wrisley DM, Whitney SL, Furman JM (2002) Vestibular rehabilitation outcomes in patients with a history of migraine. Otol Neurotol 23(4):483–487

Cervical Vertigo/Labyrinthitis/Ototoxicity

6

Many populations in the world are growing grey. Major economies are under severe stress and strain due to the rapid fall in working age groups. Britain has an ageing population. Arthritis is a major issue here. One of the causes of vertigo in the elderly is the symptomatic factor of cervical osteoarthritis and cervical spondylosis. It is a common observation in such patients that they would complain of aches and pains at the root of the neck and shoulders. Associated with the neck pains is the symptom of positional vertigo. It is usually the extension of the neck on the lower part of the cervical spine that seems to initiate the attack, which may be momentary and usually improves with the resumption of the head posture to the normal anatomical position. Sometimes the attack of vertigo may be quite intense and may frighten the patient with its volatility and intensity.

Cervical spondylitis is a fairly common condition, which causes aches and pains in the neck and shoulders. Sometimes the patient may present with pains radiating around the neck. It may well be due to the neck position, while asleep, that may compress the nerve roots emerging out of the spondylotic vertebrae, a condition called cervical radiculitis. It may contribute to dizziness due to restricted neck movement along with stiffness and discomfort at the root of the neck.

Sloane et al. (1989) mention that cervical osteoarthritis is the commonest cause of impairment of the neck proprioceptive function.

The functional control of balance rests with the central nervous system, which is loyally supported by proprioceptive impulses arriving from different bodily parts. In cervical osteoarthritis they are affected, hence contributing to imbalance and disequilibrium.

One essential investigation in these patients prior to requesting for VFT is to arrange for a CT scan of the neck. The scans have all but replaced the plain view of the neck in anteroposterior and a lateral position. More often than not, it should show degenerative changes in the vertebral bodies with lipping and sometimes bony thickening along the anterior cervical ligament. In such patients, physiotherapy is usually helpful in the control of dizziness. The important differential diagnosis, of course, is the BPPV.

S.H. Zaidi, A. Sinha, *Vertigo*,
DOI 10.1007/978-3-642-36485-3_6, © Springer-Verlag Berlin Heidelberg 2013

It is a diagnostic of elimination in many cases, particularly if the subject is young without a definite history of aches and pains in the neck or upper torso.

Such patient may not be referred for vestibulometry, particularly bitherbal calorimetry. Due to restricted neck movements, any manoeuvre such as the Dix–Hallpike test or any other form of head rotation test must be avoided, or it may precipitate acute pain and even more serious complications.

In fact, the diagnosis of cervicogenic vertigo is simple and clinical. Once again, we emphasise the value of history in a case of vertigo. Sometimes, however, there may be other causes of vertigo besides cervical pathology. Such are the cases where further investigations may be indicated.

6.1   Vestibular Neuronitis

It is a benign clinical condition, which is fairly common, and often seen in both young and elderly patients. The epidemiological studies conducted by Nehauser and Lampert have shown that the balance may remain affected in 30 % of the people following this viral condition Nehauser and Lampert (2009).

The key signs and symptoms of vestibular neuritis are rotatory vertigo with an acute onset lasting several days, horizontal spontaneous nystagmus (with a rotational component) towards the unaffected ear, a pathologic head impulse test towards the affected ear, a deviation of the subjective visual vertical towards the affected ear, postural imbalance with falls towards the affected ear and nausea. The head impulse test and caloric irrigation show an ipsilateral deficit of the vestibulo-ocular reflex. Vestibular neuritis is the third commonest cause of peripheral vestibular vertigo. It has an annual incidence of 3.5 per 100,000 population and accounts for 7 % of the patients at outpatient clinics specialising in the treatment of vertigo. The reactivation of a latent herpes simplex virus type 1 (HSV-1) infection is the most likely cause, as HSV-1 DNA and RNA have been detected in the human vestibular ganglia. Vestibular neuritis is a diagnosis of exclusion. Relevant differential diagnoses are vestibular pseudo-neuritis due to acute pontomedullary brainstem lesions or cerebellar nodular infarctions, vestibular migraine and mono-symptomatic Meniere's disease. Recovery from vestibular neuritis is due to a combination of (a) peripheral restoration of labyrinthine function, usually incomplete but can be improved by early treatment with corticosteroids, which cause a recovery rate of 62 % within 12 months; (b) mainly somatosensory and visual substitution; and (c) central compensation, which can be improved by vestibular exercise.

The exact aetiology remains unknown; as mentioned in a study quoted earlier, the viruses are often blamed for the causation. It is often preceded by a bout of flu or bad head cold. The first experience of the attack is not only crippling but also highly demoralising for the patient. Literally out of the blue, a volatile bout of vertigo with nausea and vomiting hits the patient almost randomly. Having no knowledge nor indeed a previous experience of the volatile vertigo, unlike patient of Meniere's, this patient becomes extremely worried for his life, often mistaking it for a brain haemorrhage, paralysis or a stroke.

Typically, a patient of vestibular neuritis wakes up in the middle of the night, with an acute and volatile vertigo, with the room spinning and everything going topsy-turvy. It has been described as the feeling of the sinking Titanic or at least the walk on the starboard deck of a cruise ship on a windy day. Panic stricken, gasping for breath more out of fear than actual dyspnoea, perspiring and sweating and unable to maintain his balance, the patient calls the ambulance service and is taken to the hospital. The fear of life either it being a heart attack or a stroke is certainly the main worry at this time. In due course of time, the condition settles down, and dizziness is gradually replaced with momentary postural imbalance. Other symptoms also settle down and the relief to the patient is immense. In the entire episode, there is not the slightest of involvement of haring and often enough even tinnitus is absent, though it can be noticed by some patients. Obviously, with the overbearing anxiety and severe depression at the first experience of intense vertigo can be the possible explanation of tinnitus, the cochlear component of the 8th cranial nerve escapes, and the damage is selectively confined to the vestibular part. That has been the reason why some people think it may not be a super-selective virus but just a spasm in the vascular supply of the vestibular nerve.

The condition is, fortunately, self-limiting and is seldom, if ever repeated, in the same patient. The diagnosis is mainly clinical. The main differential diagnosis being the epidemic labyrinthitis, Meniere's and transient ischemia (TIA). History has a major role to play in systematically eliminating more sinister causes of acute vertiginous symptoms. During the attack, neither audiological nor vestibular investigations are recommended. Later on, the standard protocol for detailed audio-vestibular investigation is applied.

Recently, research has been directed towards the diagnostic application of vestibular-evoked myogenic potentials. Curthoys and colleagues (2009) remind us that the bone-conducted vibration of the head causes linear acceleration stimulation of both inner ears. The same principle as applied to the time honoured Weber's tuning fork test. This liner acceleration is an effective way of selectively activating otolith afferent neurons. This simple stimulus is used to evaluate the function of the otolith bodies, clinically. A myogenic potential called n10 is evaluated through a sensitive test. In patients with total unilateral superior vestibular neuritis with intact saccular function, but the vestibular function largely compromised, the response to n10 is seen to reduce beneath the contralateral eye, strongly indicating that n10 is due to utricular otolith function (Curthoys et al. 2009). Utricle as we know is one of the essential focal points in maintenance of head posture in relation to gravity.

This test is still being developed by the scientists and may soon prove to be an essential diagnostic tool in vestibular neuritis.

Vertiginous patients often recover well from viral afflictions, but some may have protracted recovery requiring rehabilitative measures. Badaracco et al. (2007)

investigated the outcomes in chronic vertiginous patients through computerised dynamic visual acuity.

They evaluated the efficiency of the rehabilitative protocols in patients with reduced labyrinthine function, focusing on computerised dynamic visual acuity test (DVAt) and gaze stabilisation test (GST), specifically evaluating the vestibulo-oculomotor reflex (VOR) changes due to vestibular rehabilitation.

It was noted that the patients significantly improved in all the tests, thereby concluding that the vestibular rehabilitation improved the quality of life by reducing the handicap index and improving the ability in everyday tasks.

If one can improve the daily output of these patients so that they became less reliant on help, one would feel satisfied with the task performed.

Acute vestibular neuritis is a crippling condition; however, if the viral affliction is mild, it may not cause severe symptoms and may often mimic BPPV or indeed be masked by the latter.

Zapala et al. (2006) reported that a 47-year-old woman presented to the emergency department with an acute vertigo. She was diagnosed to have simultaneous acute left labyrinthitis and left posterior canal benign paroxysmal positional vertigo (BPPV). On routine clinical examination, it was also observed that gaze nystagmus from labyrinthitis hampered diagnosis of the BPPV. However, once the BPPV was identified and treated, the patient's subjective vertigo improved rapidly. This study informs us that concomitant BPPV should not be overlooked when a diagnosis of acute labyrinthitis is made in the emergency department.

Case Report

P who was born in the 1940s was referred to our vestibular lab, where she was investigated in 2011. P reported that in December 2010 she experienced a horrible attack of rotatory vertigo as she tried to lift her head and turn to her right in the middle of the night. She was frightened and kept still, lying on her back waiting for her dizziness to disappear. But it did not and persisted for 3 days. She was thus bed bound for those miserable few days. Lifting the head or suddenly moving it to one side exacerbated her dizziness even now. Therefore, she tended to restrict her head movements, specially avoiding a movement to turn to the left. She also complained of arthritis in the neck and said that even normal eye and head movement made her feel dizzy.

She had no history of hearing loss or tinnitus. There was nothing of significance in her ENT history either.

Her otoscopy was normal, and tympanometry indicated normal middle ear functions bilaterally. A PTA recorded a few days earlier was also normal.

On functional testing, Mrs. P was able to maintain her balance when reliant on her vestibular input. She failed to perform a sharpened Romberg's test with eyes closed, but Utenberger test revealed no significant rotation. Clinical rotating chair provoked good and essentially equal responses following a left and right rotation. Ocular motor testing using VNG did not reveal any abnormalities of saccades or smooth pursuit eye movements. There was no spontaneous gaze-evoked or rebound nystagmus. Dix–Hallpike testing was negative on the right and positive on the left. Calorimetry was fixed for a later date.

Her history was highly suggestive of labyrinthitis with secondary BPPV. A modified Epley's manoeuvre was performed on the left side, and a follow-up appointment was given for calorimetry as well as vestibular rehab exercises.

6.2 Viral Labyrinthitis

It is commonly seen during the cold winter months, though it may be experienced in other seasons too. It is said to be viral in origin and mimics vestibular neuronitis rather closely. The major difference is the involvement of the cochlear component in viral labyrinthitis. Vestibular neuronitis typically should not have involvement of the auditory component. In other words, there should be vertigo without a concomitant hearing loss.

Viral labyrinthitis may affect any age but is commonly seen in the aged and the immune-compromised subjects or people with ill health. Obviously, immunity plays a role in these and many similar viral infections.

A typical episode hits the patient like a tsunami. Intense degree of vertigo which is literally crippling associated with vasovagal symptoms like nausea, sickness, sweating and even pallor may be seen. Besides, the most worrying thing for the patient is the loss of hearing which is unilateral and could vary from moderate to profound and even total loss. It is associated with deafening tinnitus, again unilateral and insomniac in nature. So the overall picture is that of misery and much grief. Bilateral labyrinthitis is unusual, but can happen, when it is absolutely devastating for the sufferer. A possible underlying factor of co-morbidity such as diabetes or immune-compromised status may have a role to play in such cases.

The clinical picture may vary between the patients and can be fleeting in nature in some but more volatile and morbid in many others. The loss of hearing that has protracted prognosis takes a long time to recover, but balance improves in a few weeks and that in itself is quite reassuring.

The acute stage may last a few weeks and usually rest and simple labyrinthine sedatives suffice, but audio-vestibular tests should be requested after the acute attack is over.

Severe bilateral labyrinthitis is a horrible experience and may incapacitate the patient for a long, long time. Vertigo may gradually settle down, with the help of anti-vertiginous drugs as well as physical rehabilitation therapy, but the hearing loss could be intense and permanent (Fig. 6.1). Hearing aids may be helpful in most but not in all cases. In profound cases of post-labyrinthitis hearing impairment, hearing therapy may be helpful. In some cases of total deafness, language therapy may be the final rehab alternative. Such patients should be referred to a special otology centre for assessment regarding a cochlear implant.

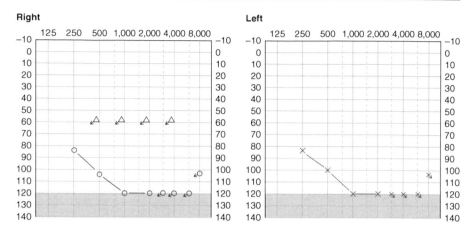

Fig. 6.1 This pure tone audiogram (PTA) shows bilateral profound sensorineural hearing loss, following a severe bout of labyrinthitis in an extremely unusual case. Hearing did not return, but vertigo settled down after intensive treatment and rehab therapy. Even a hearing aid was not helpful. Hearing therapy was advised. In some patients, a cochlear implant may be an option

6.3   Vestibular Compensation

An acute attack of vertigo such as caused by vestibular neuritis obviously is the result of an insult or injury to the vestibular organ. Soon after, however, the CNS takes up the responsibility of bring about compensation. The compensatory process is usually slow and may vary from person to person as indeed the cause of vestibulopathy. Some may recover faster than others.

It is believed that at rest the sensory hair cells in semicircular canals, the utricle and the saccule have a tonic firing rate. Each sense organ has contralateral sensory organ to correspond with the anatomical site. The semicircular canals, for instance, have a prearranged relationship with the opposite ear. When a side is traumatised, the impulses are slowed down, but the vestibular nuclei take over the function by increasing the firing rate on the traumatised side while diminishing the firing rate on the unaffected side so that a state of balance is achieved. It is a natural physiological phenomenon, which must be allowed to continue. Drug-induced return of balance after an acute episode of vertigo delays the compensation mechanism by disturbing the physiology. It is therefore the best practice to prescribe anti-vertiginous drugs only for a brief period and allow the natural vestibular compensation to take place.

6.4   Motion Sickness/Travel Sickness

It is an extremely common entity. Anyone who has experienced a voyage on a boat, short or long, in a choppy sea may have experienced it. The intensity of dizziness and associated symptoms like nausea and vomiting may vary from person to person.

People who have a rather susceptible labyrinth may even feel vertiginous in a moving car or a ride in a lift. As a matter of fact, it is a hypersensitivity of the vestibular system rather than a significant pathology that initiates the symptoms. The best treatment of course is in avoidance of the precipitating causes like a boat trip or a ride on merry go round, let alone the speedy topsy-turvy theme park rides. Hyoscine dermal patch is known to be effective in most patients and does not require being plastered on the mastoid bone. The dermal penetration will take place from any part of the body any way, but it is a common practice to apply the patch closer to the ear, which may indeed have an added psychological advantage.

6.5   Perilymph Fistula

It is an uncommon condition that may affect any age group, but most often younger folks. It has no underlying cause nor indeed any definite explanation. It may however be preceded by either a robust physical exercise or a strain. The hypothesis is that either due to excessive increase in the perilymph content or indeed natural weakness or dehiscence of the labyrinthine capsule, the perilymph leaks out, causing severe vertigo, nausea and vomiting, hearing loss, tinnitus, etc. Round window rupture syndrome has been described in the textbooks as one similar condition with a natural dehiscence of the round window or a fragile secondary tympanic membrane that bursts under undue physical pressure and may cause acute symptoms of vertigo mimicking labyrinthitis.

Following the stapes surgery, perilymph leak is a common observation and is the underlying reason for post-stapedectomy dizziness. It settles down in due course of time without the need of many drugs. One of the main tell-tale signs of having achieved successful removal of the whole or a part of the footplate of stapes is the appearance of a fine and thin layer of clear perilymph at the site of perforation with the 'pick'. Sometimes, a portion of the footplate would become lose and refractory to extraction. We did not unduly attempt to remove this so-called floating footplate, as cases were reported when an aggressive surgeon chasing the wobbly footplate ended up with a dead ear. In fact, stapes surgery was best performed under local infiltration anaesthesia and mild sedation. Those of us who performed these surgeries in the past decades were unusually gratified with the spontaneous joy of a 'deaf' person returning from the operating room clearly hearing the faintest of sounds, which he may never have heard before.

A fateful moment can bring about a revolution. That is what happened when John Shea who performed the first ever stapedectomy revolutionised the management of otosclerosis forever. But earlier on, many masters like Brownly Smith, Mcleod and Macklay and surely many more were performing a highly skilled operation to relieve the problem of hearing impairment caused by otosclerosis. It was called the 'fenestration'. It literally involved creating a new window in the lateral or horizontal semicircular canal, with a view to bypass the fixed stapes and transfer the sound through this third window in the inner ear. They would drill the bone to such thinness that the 'bluish hue' of the membranous labyrinth would show like a silhouette. It was a masterly technique and dedicated to a few centres only. The patient would resume his hearing, following a fenestration procedure, albeit felt perpetually unsteady on his feet. Rarely, this procedure would cause a perilymph leak, requiring its closure and abandoning of the fenestration.

Acute spontaneous perilymph leak may sometimes require exploratory tympan-otomy and closure of the fistula employing a blob of fat or an autogenous material to plug the leak. It is rare but has to be kept in mind as a differential diagnosis in cases of post-traumatic vertigo.

Banerjee and colleagues (2005) mentioned an unusual cause of vertigo, which may fall into the differential diagnosis of a perilymph fistula, or a round window rupture syndrome.

They called this new cause of sound- and pressure-induced vertigo 'superior canal dehiscence'. They noted that auditory manifestations of this unusual condi-tion include hyperacusis to bone-conducted sounds and conductive hearing loss with normal acoustic reflexes. The diagnosis was reached by a directed history, documentation of upward and torsional nystagmus evoked by sound and pressure, and radiology. Acoustic reflexes and VEMP (vestibular-evoked myogenic poten-tials) were employed as an aid in the identification of patients with an apparent conductive loss with normal acoustic reflexes or who had an asymptomatic dehis-cence proven radiologically. The treatment involved the avoidance of the precipitat-ing stimuli. They also recommended surgical treatment, by resurfacing the dehiscence, in patients with severe symptoms.

One must remember that it is an unusual condition. We have no experience in dealing with this problem surgically, and there are not many reports available to commend the procedure without further studies.

6.6   Ototoxicity

There are many drugs that are known to be ototoxic. A group of antibiotics called the aminoglycosides deserve to be mentioned as the most potent of them all. Streptomycin has been in use since the end of the second war and has indeed proved to be a panacea in tuberculosis. In the developing countries where TB has been rampant for millennia, streptomycin has saved hundreds of thousands of lives and continues to do so. However, its side effects particularly tinnitus, cochlear damage and vertigo have been tolerated as a small price to pay for a life-saving drug. Vestibular toxicity is one of the reasons that many physicians are obliged to discon-tinue the therapy while the full course still remains to be completed. Sensorineural hearing loss and tinnitus are sometimes, but not always, equal contenders in the process of abandoning the drug mid-therapy.

Gentamicin is another drug that can easily take to its credit many cases of ves-tibular toxicity. It is a powerful antibiotic and often enough genuine life saver, but it is highly ototoxic. In fact in some patients its use is so inevitable that a minor price of ototoxicity is duly ignored by the physicians. In patients with chronic renal disease where gentamicin is often indicated for combating septicaemia, the prognosis of ototoxicity is even worse. Not only because these patients have poor glomerular filtration rate but also the fact that some of them are on loop diuretics, which in their own right are highly ototoxic. Gentamicin is also used as a potent medico-surgical treatment for chronic uncontrollable Meniere's disease, if the cochlear function is already compromised.

The topical use of gentamicin in actively discharging ears may be forgiven as the local absorption, though the mucosa of the promontory may not be sufficient enough to cause vestibular damage, but in a dry perforation, it may be avoided as the concentration may rise due to the lack of the dilution effect of otorrhoea.

Other aminoglycosides often used in some cases are amikacin, tobramycin, neomycin, framycetin, soframycin and kanamycin. One important non-aminoglycoside antibiotic belonging to macrolide group is erythromycin which can be ototoxic in a small number of cases.

We were asked to monitor the progress of hearing in a young man on amikacin for a systemic infection. He certainly showed a drop in some frequencies, after a few weeks of treatment, so we had to recommend to his physician to reduce the dose and, if possible, discontinue the amikacin. Soon after, we checked him again to note that hearing loss had stabilised. Regrettably, the drop in hearing was sensorineural.

As mentioned before, loop diuretics like furosemides, bumetanide and ethacrynic acid are another important group of drugs that are known to cause ototoxicity. In a patient who may have highly compromised renal function, the cumulative effect of loop diuretics may result in marked ototoxicity. The early appearance of vertiginous symptoms in such patients is a warning sign for withholding the drugs. Many renal and cardiac failure patients who often need the loop diuretics are immune compromised also and require repeated courses of antibiotics. The problem of vestibulocochlear ototoxicity multiplies manifold in such patients if they are given the aminoglycoside while on loop diuretics.

Amongst the other more important drugs that a clinician may encounter in daily practice, one has to remember the beta blockers and calcium channel blockers which are known to cause dizziness. A cardiac patient, who may have postural hypotension or indeed angina causing light-headedness, should always be checked for potential contributors like the blockers mentioned before.

Chemotherapy plays an invaluable role in the management of many malignancies. Some of them are highly ototoxic and would require auditory and vestibular monitoring. Cisplatin is one important chemotherapeutic drug often employed in the treatment of many head and neck cancers. Carboplatin is another potentially ototoxic drug often used in cancer chemotherapy with potential risks of ototoxicity, particularly in children. The main ototoxic effect of course is irreversible hearing loss, which is usually related to the cumulative dosage and interaction with concomitant medical therapy such as the use of aminoglycoside.

Now uncommon in UK but in malaria-ridden countries, quinine remains a common cause of vertigo. It is currently being used for the treatment of leg cramps, and if the patient feels vertiginous, it may be the appropriate time to stop quinine.

As an example of vestibular damage caused by drugs, the following report of two cases of unilateral vestibulopathies after systemic ototoxic treatment is mentioned here Martinez J and Rey-Martinez (2005).

The patients were seen after having recovered from their initial illnesses, and both of them denied suffering any spells of vertigo, loss of hearing during the treatment or tinnitus. In both patients, oscillopsia and vestibular ataxia were of varying intensity. Bedside vestibular examination, caloric and rotatory chair testing and vestibular-evoked myogenic potentials were congruent with a complete unilateral loss of vestibular function. Audiometry was normal in one case, but in the other, there was a moderate bilateral sensorineural loss of hearing that was present before treatment and that did not change during the course of the treatment. It was concluded that the existence of unilateral vestibular loss was an unsuspected finding, but after careful bedside examination, it was confirmed through extensive vestibular testing.

References

Badaracco C, Labini FS, Meli A, De Angelis E, Tufarelli D (2007) Vestibular rehabilitation outcomes in chronic vertiginous patients through computerized dynamic visual acuity and Gaze stabilization test. Otol Neurotol 28(6):809–813, 1531–7129

Banerjee A, Whyte A, Atlas MD (2005) Superior canal dehiscence: review of a new condition. Clin Otolaryngol 30(1):9–15, 1749–4478

Curthoys IS, Manzari L, Smulders YE, Burgess AM (2009) A review of the scientific basis and practical application of a new test of utricular function – ocular vestibular-evoked myogenic potentials to bone-conducted vibration. Acta Otolaryngol Ital 29(4):179–186, 0392–100X; 1827–675X

Martinez J, Rey-Martinez J, Rama-Lopez J, Soledad Boleas M, Perez N, Artieda J (2005) Deux cas de vestibulopathie unilatérale après traitement ototoxique systémique. Rev Laryngol Otol Rhinol 126(3):159–163, 0035–1334

Nehauseur HK, Lampert T (2009) Vestibular neuritis. Semin Neurol 29(5):509–519, 0271–8235; 1098–9021

Slaone P, Blazer D, George L (1989) Dizziness in a community elderly population. J Am Geriatr Soc 37(2):101–108

Zapala DA, Shapiro SA, Lundy LB, Leming DT (2006) Simultaneous acute superior nerve neuro-labyrinthitis and benign paroxysmal positional vertigo. J Am Acad Audiol 17(7):481–486; quiz 531–532, 1050–0545

Chronic Suppurative Otitis Media (CSOM)

7

Textbooks are full of the description of chronic supportive otitis media, its aetiology, pathology, complications and management. We have included salient clinical features here.

By definition, otitis media is an inflammatory condition that involves the lining membrane of the middle ear cleft. Embryologically, this cleft develops from the second branchial arch and comprises of three components, namely, the Eustachian tube, the middle ear and the mastoid process. The process of inflammation in otitis media may therefore involve all three structures but must remain confined to the lining epithelium only. The moment this infection exceeds the confines of the epithelium, such as the mastoid bone, it ceases to be called an otitis media and is usually labelled a complication such as mastoiditis or petrositis. Mastoid abscess, facial paralysis, meningitis Gradinego's syndrome, etc. were fairly known complications of the past.

There are two types of chronic middle ear infections, namely, the mucoid or nonsuppurative and the suppurative otitis media. It is the chronic suppurative otitis media that may be a cause of vertigo in some patients. We shall therefore concentrate on the discussion on CSOM only. The nonsuppurative form of chronic suppurative otitis media is primarily a mucosal disease, involving the mucosa of the mesotympanum and hypotympanum. It does not usually lead to complications such as labyrinthitis. It is, however, responsible for causing conductive form of hearing impairment (Fig. 7.1). It is also called the 'safe type of CSOM'. In children, it is a fairly common cause of hearing impairment, described as the 'glue ear'. Relief is easily and briskly achieved through a myringotomy and grommet/ventilation tube insertion, albeit not without some possible side effects like a nonhealing perforation.

The second form is more relevant to our subject. It involves the attic part of the middle ear and may lead to complications like labyrinthitis. It is sometimes described as an 'unsafe type of CSOM'. It may be unilateral or bilateral and leads to marked conductive hearing loss as seen in this audiogram (Fig. 7.2).

S.H. Zaidi, A. Sinha, *Vertigo*,
DOI 10.1007/978-3-642-36485-3_7, © Springer-Verlag Berlin Heidelberg 2013

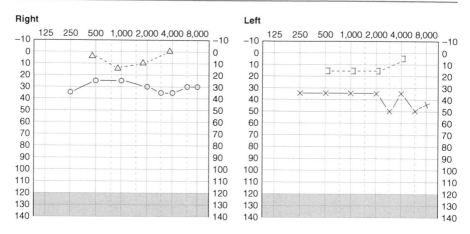

Fig. 7.1 This audiogram shows an air-bone gap in a case of chronic (mucoid) nonsuppurative otitis media. The air conduction is markedly less than bone conduction across the range of frequencies between 250 and 8,000 Hz, indicative of conductive hearing loss brought about by effusion in the middle ears

The hallmark of the so-called unsafe CSOM is the presence of a substance called cholesteatoma, within the middle ear cavity. So much research has been conducted on the subject of cholesteatoma that in the decades of 1970s, the academicians had to hold international meetings dedicated only to cholesteatoma. It was a major cause of concern to the otologists in the world over for at least half a century if not more. The good news is that its incidence and prevalence have significantly dropped globally, albeit still a common cause of intracranial complications in many developing countries.

Cholesteatoma is a keratinous material that is a by-product of desquamation of the squamous epithelium in the middle ear. And that is a million dollar question. Since the epithelium of the middle ear is basically cuboidal in the epitympanum or attic area and columnar in the meso- and hypotympanum, how does one explain the appearance of cholesteatoma as a by-product of squamous epithelium at a site where normally there is no squamous epithelium? Volumes have been written on the hypotheses of the possible explanation for this phenomenon. The reader is advised to benefit from such masterly treatises for further enlightenment on the origin of cholesteatoma. The most plausible explanation is the process of metaplasia brought about by subminimal inflammation, in the epitympanum, converting the cuboidal into squamous epithelium. This squamous epithelium in turn leads to the development of cholesteatoma. Proponents of the theory of Eustachian tube dysfunction claim that the whole process of low-grade inflammation described above can be prevented by the insertion of grommet. They therefore claim that the decline in the incidence of cholesteatoma began with the introduction of myringotomy and grommet insertion in the late 1970s, which is possibly true.

This keratinous material which looks and feels like a poultice, fairly innocuous in form and texture, may sometimes bring about a havoc in the middle ear. It has been known and seen to cause serious and life-threatening complication like

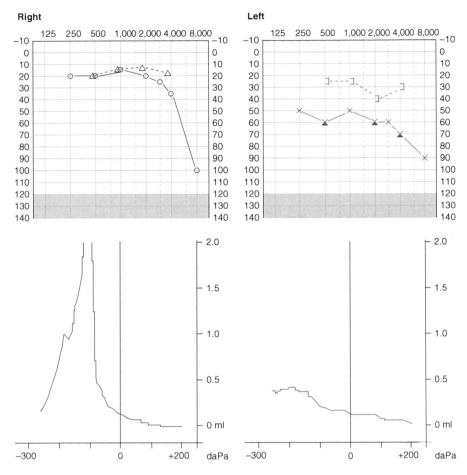

Fig. 7.2 A pure tone audiogram (PTA) showing conductive hearing loss in the left ear caused by CSOM with cholesteatoma. The hearing level in the right ear is normal in the speech range. The *lower part* of this figure shows a type C tympanogram in the left ear, due to an attic retraction of the tympanic membrane. Right ear shows a type Ad tympanogram due to hypermobility

meningitis, extradural abscess subdural abscess, a temporal lobe abscess, lateral sinus thrombosis, otitic hydrocephalus and of course labyrinthitis, a subject that concerns us most. Facial nerve paralysis was often the first sign of impending complications in those days.

As a matter of fact, some of the ENT surgeons had the opportunity of dealing with the serious intracranial complications of cholesteatoma in the early part of their careers. Those who practised in the developing countries had to drain the brain abscesses resulting from invasion of cholesteatoma, let alone dealing with common but less threatening problems like meningitis and extradural abscesses.

It is said that cholesteatoma has an inherent capacity to release certain catabolic enzymes with osteolytic potency, which may be responsible for eroding the middle ear ossicles, eating away the thick and sturdy tegmen tympani which isolates the brain from the attic region of the middle ear. As it is beyond the scope of this book, the reader is best advised to benefit from the textbooks regarding the mode of action of cholesteatoma in causing demolition of the middle ear contents as well as the neighbouring structures.

Labyrinthitis is a known complication of CSOM. Cholesteatoma literally erodes away the otic capsule to cause the symptoms of acute sometimes chronic relapsing vertigo. In fact, if a patient with known history of chronic discharging ear begins to develop vertigo, it is an absolute indicator that there may be more than the superficial mucosal disease in the middle ear.

The CT scan has changed the picture altogether. It may show the erosion of the labyrinthine capsule or a massive cholesteatoma encroaching onto the neighbouring structures. A CT scan in cases of CSOM presenting with an attic retraction pocket, or a pouch; or the telltale signs of middle ear pathology, a featureless, colourless, bulging eardrum; or a polyp or granulation tissue in the pars flaccida is absolutely necessary and may indeed prove to be a life-saver.

One can never show enough gratitude to the colleagues in the radiology department to guide us in such situations. Sometimes, however, a clinician may prefer to wait and watch, even though the CT shows a cholesteatoma. This usually applies to small and lazy cholesteatoma, in such an ear, which is called a 'quiet ear'. It means that the potential danger of activity may still exist, just like a sleeping volcano, but there may not be any urgency in intervening in the ear just yet. Watchful waiting may be the suitable also in some patients where the ear has been discharging but has now settled down.

Natural healing is known to happen in the middle ears just as elsewhere in the body. The disease dies away or simply 'burns' itself out.

An important clinical test for possible involvement of the labyrinth in CSOM is called the fistula test. By deliberately raising and releasing the pressure in the outer ear canal of the suspected side either manually or with a siegel's pneumatic speculum, one asks the patient for dizziness while simultaneously checking for nystagmus. If the patient feels giddy and the nystagmus is noticed, then it is labelled as a 'positive fistula test'. It is also called a Hennebert's sign. It is an indicator of involvement of the labyrinth due to a possible erosion of the bony labyrinthine capsule by cholesteatoma (Fig. 7.3).

Beside cholesteatoma, there could be many other causes for the development a perilymph fistula. Some of these are barotrauma, acoustic trauma, congenital malformation of the Mondini type, congenital, superior canal dehiscence, jugular dehiscence, iatrogenic such as after cochlear implants, or a combined approach tympanoplasty (CAT), mastoid surgery, tympanoplasty, intratympanic facial nerve surgery, spontaneous idiopathic round window rupture syndrome and vestibulofibrosis.

The clinical diagnosis of a perilymph fistula can therefore be challenging, but detailed history and proper diagnostic tests including imaging should establish the real cause of the fistula.

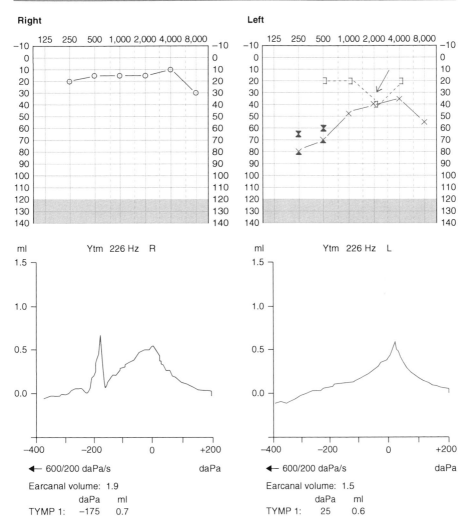

Fig. 7.3 This Audiogram shows conductive hearing loss in the left ear, due to middle ear disease. Both tympanograms are normal with a possible artefact on the right side

CSOM is known to cause many other complications such as facial paralysis, labyrinthitis or even brain abscess. Suffice it to say that when dealing with a case of cholesteatoma, one must remain on guard and investigate the patient thoroughly, particularly through a CT scan. Not all patients may require surgery, as sometimes the CSOM may burn itself out. Watchful waiting is the usual practice in such situations; however, if the patient remains asymptomatic for a long duration, he may be discharged.

Many mastoid cavities require an aural toilet. Some patients may feel dizzy following such a procedure. It is usually momentarily brought about by stimulation of an otherwise normal labyrinth. In the early days of the mastoid surgery before reputedly Simpson Hall introduced the microscope to ENT surgery, and before the advent of electric drills, such a surgery was often performed by masters employing a head mirror and hammer and gouge. There were many problems, but the surgeons had acquired suitable skills through hard work and dedication. Despite that, a CSF leak would sometimes appear as the chisel could damage the thin tegmen tympani. Such patients would develop acute vertigo and progressively worsening headache, a clear sign of impending meningitis. Many a times, in order to clear out the cholesteatoma obsessively, surgeons would drill the mastoid bowl so thin that the lateral semicircular canal would become almost skeletonised. Such a patient would often experience vertigo on the slightest exposure of the affected ear to a stimulus, as imperceptible as a gentle breeze. Those early ear surgeons were obsessed with cholesteatoma because they had seen people dying of brain abscess brought about by the erosion of the roof of the middle ear by an aggressive cholesteatoma.

Most cavities stabilise over time and do not require a follow-up. Some cavities may grow narrower and smaller and require no more than the usual care and protection from external contamination.

Those days are gone when large cavities leading to repeated infections demanded closure or obliteration through pedicled grafts or fancier techniques employing bone pate etc. The character and the size of the cavities also depend upon the race and morphological features of a skull. This subject was studied anthropologically by Zaidi, a few years ago (1989). Morphological features of the skull, head and neck, indeed the whole human body, may sometimes help explain a few causes of vertigo. For instance, the Asian neck is rather pliable and very flexible, which may be a factor in hypothesising that cervicogenic vertigo is less common in them than the Alpine and Celtic races. An illustration of cervical flexibility could be noted in an Indian dancing girl, who can move her neck horizontally along the C8–T1 vertebral joint, adding further glamour to her dancing prowess.

As the technology advanced, maestros of ear surgery like Fisch, Sheehy, Paparella, Potmannan and Smyth (just to mention a few names) and many other otologists developed even finer techniques which would avoid the creation of a mastoid bowl, without compromising the safety of the patient by totally eradicating the cholesteatoma. Furthermore, they could also repair the functional damage caused by the disease or its surgical management, simultaneously by performing a single stage or later on as a two-staged tympanoplasty. This technique is called an intact wall tympanoplasty or combined approach tympanoplasty (CAT). It is still in vogue, but due to the overall decline in the prevalence of cholesteatoma, it is practised less often now than before.

Reference

Zaidi SH (1989) An anthropological study of the mastoid air cell system in skulls. J Laryngol Otol
      103:819–822

Central Causes

8

8.1   Acoustic Neuroma

Acoustic neuroma is a benign, slow-growing tumour arising from the specialised cells of the eighth cranial nerve. These cells are called the Schwann cells. Hence, the tumour is sometimes called a schwannoma. They can occur elsewhere in the body too, as was our experience quite recently.

We saw this lady who had a schwannoma removed from her lung and was referred to us for investigation of the possible coexistence of schwannoma in the eighth nerve. An MRI scan was requested which was reported negative. Apparently similar cases have been found and reported in China and elsewhere too. A total of 40 schwannoma are reported in the literature, which are found to originate in sites other than the inner ear.

Acoustic neuromas originate within the internal auditory canal and slowly find their way out of the internal auditory meatus to occupy the cerebellopontine angle. Initially the symptoms may be mild such as unilateral tinnitus or sensorineural hearing loss but could get worse as the tumour progresses.

Balance is initially not affected, though sometimes patient may feel unsteady on feet. However, as the tumour becomes extra-canalicular and engages the cerebello-pontine structures, symptoms may vary from the trigeminal nerve involvement to acute ataxia. The facial nerve is sitting isolated from the vestibulocochlear nerve in the internal meatus, but an expanding tumour can encroach upon it resulting in ipsilateral facial nerve paralysis, an extremely unpleasant sign indeed.

It is always an essential differential diagnosis in a case of unilateral symptoms of vertigo, tinnitus and unilateral or asymmetrical sensorineural hearing loss (Fig. 8.1).

In many cases of bilateral symptoms also, an acoustic neuroma may require to be excluded. Of course, being a highly specialised pathology, it is not expected that every ENT surgeon should be able to handle them. It is, however, expected that every ENT person should be able to pick up these tumours early, diagnose them and refer the patient as early as possible to the specialised department dealing with them. There are many centres in the UK, where this precision surgery is performed by the specialist otolaryngologists and neuro-otologists.

S.H. Zaidi, A. Sinha, *Vertigo*,
DOI 10.1007/978-3-642-36485-3_8, © Springer-Verlag Berlin Heidelberg 2013

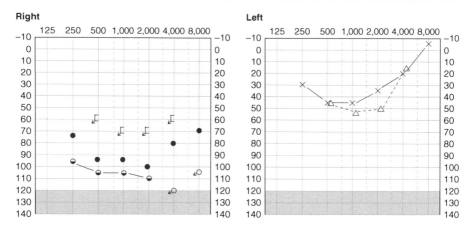

Fig. 8.1 The audiogram showing asymmetrical sensorineural hearing loss. The hearing loss is severe to profound in intensity (above 85 dB) in the right ear and mild to moderate (40–60 dB) in the left ear. This is an audiogram of a case of suspected acoustic neuroma in the right ear, requiring scanning and neurological opinion

History and clinical diagnosis must follow detailed investigations in a suspected acoustic neuroma. An MRI and detailed audio-vestibular investigation are mandatory in these cases. We employ VNG as a diagnostic tool to help us identify a central pathology in a multitude of causes of vertigo. An illustration of such a VNG tracing is included in the chapter on VNGs in this book (Fig. 2.1).

The incidence of schwannoma has been the subject of many studies. Mirko Tos was an otologist of outstanding repute. He did many pioneering works in this field in Scandinavia. Tos et al. (1999) investigated the incidence of acoustic neuromas in Denmark over a period of several years. It was a retrospective review of prospective registered data on all patients with VS operated on by the translabyrinthine, lateral suboccipital or middle cranial fossa approach, as well as patients who were allocated to the 'wait-and-scan' group. Patient's charts were reviewed and tabulated for age, extrameatal tumour extension and date of diagnosis. The available data was divided into three periods. A significant increase in incidence of the newly diagnosed intracanalicular tumours in the second and third periods was observed.

Tos therefore concluded that the increase in incidence could probably be explained by the awareness and better access to diagnostic radiology. They observed though that the increase in the diagnosis of the small and intrameatal tumour created a clinical dilemma, as to whether to operate on tumours in this early stage or to allocate patients to the wait-and-scan group. This problem will still be relevant in the upcoming years, since the incidence of intrameatal and small tumours is expected to increase.

Tos mentioned this some years ago. The universal policy nowadays is the conservative management. Since they are extremely slow-growing tumours, surgery on a minute tumour may harm the patient more than benefit. The fundamental principle of medical ethics called nonmaleficence goes hand in hand with the principle of beneficence. And this may well be a good example of observing the two basic rules of medical ethics. Surgery is still carried out, albeit only in those tumours that encroach upon the pontine–medullary axis, after exceeding the confines of the internal auditory canal.

Another important study on the incidence and prevalence of acoustic neuromas was conducted, in Denmark, by a different group (Mirz et al. 2000).

They looked at 162 tumours over a period of 21 years. They noted that there was a noticeable but gradual increase in the incidence during this period, which they suspect could be due to improvement of the quality of radiological imaging.

Their long but controlled follow-up showed that 14 tumours (22 %) regressed, 35 (55 %) did not grow or had only minimal growth (growth rate up to 1 mm/year), whereas 15 VS (23 %) grew >1 mm/year.

This invaluable study once again duly highlights the point that an acoustic neuroma is an extremely slow-growing tumour. Most people would therefore manage it on the basis of wait-and-see policy.

The following study was broad-based involving the epidemiological evaluation of primary nerve sheath tumours and its subset, i.e. acoustic neuroma Propp J.M. et al. (2006). It involved two population-based incidence registries, and data were obtained from 11 Central Brain Tumour Registry centres of the United States between 1975 and 1998. Through this highly sophisticated statistical study, the authors were able to determine that the overall incidence of primary nerve sheath tumours of the brain/CNS was 1.1 per 100,000 person-years. The incidence of vestibular schwannomas was similar for both data sets: 0.6 per 100,000 person-years and 0.8 per 100,000 person-years.

Moreover, they noted that the incidence of primary nerve sheath tumours of the brain/CNS overall and of vestibular schwannomas increased over time. However, the incidence of benign schwannomas in sites other than the acoustic nerve either decreased or experienced no significant change. The authors inferred that the trend noted was possibly due to the improvements in diagnosis and early reporting.

One essential aspect of the management of acoustic neuroma of course is its awareness and prompt diagnosis. The referral pattern of such patients who may have unexplainable symptoms like unilateral tinnitus, asymmetrical sensorineural hearing loss or vertigo to the specialist clinic is therefore an important entity.

Moffat et al. (2004) observed that the imaging techniques, awareness of pathology and prompt referral in vestibular schwannomas have all improved in the last decade.

They demonstrated an increase in the proportion of referrals with known vestibular schwannomas to 90 % of all referrals. No significant change in the length of history prior to referral or the source of referral or principal presenting symptom was found. An overall decrease in tumour size was found but an increase in the percentage with larger tumours (>4.5 cm). The authors attribute their significant findings to an increase in availability of magnetic resonance (MR) scanners in the country in the recent times. They also observed that some tumours would still present late and therefore will elude identification until large in spite of a low threshold for MR scanning.

Acoustic neuromas are investigated in many ways. The diagnostic value of vestibular-evoked myogenic potential (EMG) in patients with vestibular schwannomas was the subject of a study carried out in Japan in 2009 (Ushio et al. 2009).

This study was designed to compare the diagnostic value of VEMP in comparison with the caloric tests in patients with acoustic neuroma. The study identified that the sensitivity and specificity of the VEMPs and calorimetry showed no significant differences, highlighting that in patients with acoustic neuroma although the specificity of VEMP was not very high, its sensitivity was high and comparable to that of the calorimetry.

The tumour is best diagnosed with the help of an MRI. The importance of vestibular function tests, however, remains undiminished, as was reported in the following study (Grayeli et al. 2007).

These workers described and analysed a series of intracochlear schwannomas seen over an 8-year period. Out of the 19 positive cases, 18 had solitary tumours and 1 had neurofibromatosis type 2, which is an essential clinical entity worth keeping in mind. The diagnosis was often delayed for an average of 11 years. They employed the inevitable magnetic resonance imaging, which showed the involvement of the posterior labyrinth in eight patients (37 %), an extension of the schwannoma to the internal auditory meatus in eight patients (37 %). Even the cerebellopontine angle extension was noted in seven patients (32 %).

They observed that the diagnosis of a schwannomas can be difficult at times. MRI, however, has changed the picture and made an early diagnosis more frequent and accurate. The authors have reported a series of surgical intervention, which is interesting, as more and more otologists now diagnose a tumour early and keep them under conservative care rather than early intervention.

For many years, Manchester Royal Infirmary had a dedicated service for surgical treatment of acoustic neuromas. A pioneering surgeon, Richard Ramsden, performed many intricate surgeries on these tumours. He published extensively, and the reader may refer to his publications. In Birmingham, Richard Irving, a renowned neuro-otologist and skull base surgeon, is well known for his expertise in this field. Likewise in many other places, there are stalwarts who are continuously gaining grounds in the field of skull base surgery. By and large though, things have moved on from the early days of heroic surgery and the discovery of Bill's bar by one famous Professor Bill House to the current policy of prompt diagnosis and watchful waiting. Those who become a nuisance go under the conventional knife or a Gamma knife of the neurosurgeons or the skull base surgeons. From a routine ENT point of view, suffice it to say that the diagnosis of an acoustic neuroma must not be missed.

Case Report

P aged 68 was seen in our vestibular lab in 2010 for diagnostic tests. She described her symptoms as complete loss of balance and was indeed observed to have significant difficulty moving around the clinic. She reported that her problem began in December last year and had worsened in last 6 months or so. She reported that her first episode was noticed while at work. She lost her balance while cleaning the floors and had to hold on a neighbouring object to control her. The second attack occurred a few days later when she noted that her leg 'went to jelly' and she could not stand up to get out of the chair. Initially, similar episodes were occurring two to three times a week; however, they had now increased in frequency and intensity. She felt perpetually imbalanced. She said that before she loses her balance, she felt light-headed and for the past few weeks also had blurred vision. Making fast movements would exacerbate her symptoms. She denied any rotatory vertigo. She had constant headaches which had been attributed to a pituitary macroadenoma which was detected last December.

P said that that she had good and bad days with her balance and felt afraid of falls. She had stopped her work and usually stayed home, moving around holding objects for support.

She denied any hearing loss or tinnitus. There was no ontological history of note either. She was a migraine sufferer though the frequency of her migraine had decreased in the last few months. As an asthmatic, she used inhalers and once had a lung collapse. She also has neck and back discomfort following a slip disc approximately 16 years ago. She also reported of blurred vision and an incidence of diplopia.

No abnormalities were detected bilaterally on otoscopy, and only a mild high-frequency hearing loss bilaterally noted on audiometry. Tympanometry was normal. Upon functional testing, P was unable to maintain her balance with eyes closed. Ocular-motor testing using VNG revealed no spontaneous, gaze or rebound nystagmus. No abnormalities of saccadic or smooth pursuit eye movements were detected. She reported diplopia on several occasions while attempting to follow the target. Bithermal caloric testing revealed no significant canal paresis or directional preponderance; however, responses were hyperactive bilaterally.

It was concluded therefore that she had no evidence of a peripheral vestibular lesion. The hyperactive caloric response is unusual and suggestive of a central lesion, possibly indicating impaired inhibition within the vestibular pathway. She was already under the care of the neurology department, which was in keeping with the history and the diagnostic tests.

Case Report

P aged 58 was seen in our vestibular lab in 2010 when he said that he was unsteady on his feet, even while standing still, for the past 3–4 years. There was no sudden onset of symptoms or any noticeable event that might have initiated the problem. He became gradually aware of the need to hold on to objects when standing still. He felt the ground move under his feet, and he had to sway to maintain his balance. He could walk without feeling unsteady. He denied any rotatory vertigo but found it difficult to continue to work as teacher.

In the past, he had received chemotherapy for a cancer in 2009. Since then, he had bilateral tinnitus, aural fullness and hearing loss. There was no history of fluctuation of hearing or variation in tinnitus with the dizziness. A few months back he had developed diplopia which was attributed to an ischaemic attack. His vision had now improved with slight diplopia in his peripheral vision. Mr. P also said that he had an episode of flashing, rotary lights in his vision after a chemotherapy session, but this was not regular occurrence. He was a known hypertensive, taking ramipril. He also complained of some stiffness in the neck. He was attending outpatient clinics of oncology and neurology.

On otoscopy, everything appeared to be normal. PTA showed satisfactory hearing in both eras, with mild loss at 4 K and above. Tympanometry was normal.

Upon functional testing, Mr. P was found to be quite unsteady on his feet when vision and proprioceptive inputs were removed separately. When both vision and proprioceptive inputs were removed simultaneously, he was unable to maintain his balance. Ocular-motor testing using VNG revealed no spontaneous gaze-evoked or rebound nystagmus. Warm water screening test revealed equal and robust responses bilaterally; however, the visual fixation index was outside the normal range for both left and right beating nystagmus.

The results did not show an evidence of a peripheral vestibular pathology. Mr. P was very dependent on his visual and proprioceptive impulses to maintain his balance. The abnormal fixation index indicated an impaired ability to suppress nystagmus with fixation and may indeed be caused by a central lesion. It has been suggested that gaze stabilisation exercises may be useful for patients with central vestibular loss; hence, Mr. P would be advised accordingly through post to do the recommended exercises. It was hoped that these exercises would prove beneficial to him.

Once diagnosed, the patient should be referred to a neuro-otologist or a skull base surgeon, promptly.

8.2   Multiple Sclerosis

It is a chronic disease which is characterised by areas of demyelination, along with low-grade inflammation, and glial cicatrisation of the central nous system. It is a slowly progressive condition, varying in intensity from symptom-free periods to a disabling state.

It is an idiopathic demyelinising disorder thought to be an autoimmune in nature, most likely caused by an autoantigen to one of the myelin proteins. It is also a condition which is difficult to diagnose and treat. It is characterised by the development of pathological patches of demyelinisation in the nervous system which is followed by gliosis. Remissions are known to occur, and therefore, many times the false hope of recovery may be given to the patient. Unfortunately though, the relapses occur and can be prolonged as well as variable in intensity.

Its aetiology is unknown, and it is characterised by the widespread occurrence in the patches of demyelinisation followed by gliosis. Significant and notable improvement may sometimes give false belief of total recovery. Remissions seem to alternate with bouts of relapse. The clinical picture is one of progressive dissemination tending to produce the classic features of ataxia and disequilibrium, even paraplegia (Walton 1977).

One of the essential differential diagnoses of vertigo is the clinical entity of multiple sclerosis. It is a neurological condition and is usually seen and diagnosed by neurologists; however, a patient referred from the GP surgery with the clinical diagnosis of vertigo may require an investigation by the otolaryngologist. One essential investigation, of course, is the MRI. It is extremely helpful in the diagnosis of multiple sclerosis as indeed in other demyelinising disorders. From our point of view, we request for an MRI of the IAM and CP angle, to exclude an acoustic neuroma. Brain is usually scanned simultaneously which may show demyelinisation as the diagnosis of an MS. CSF examination is extremely helpful diagnosis as elevated levels of IgG can be identified.

Peyvandi and colleagues (2010) believe that MS can present with a variety of neurological signs and symptoms, as well as the hearing loss. They studied 30 patients of MS and carried out detailed audiological investigations including the PTA, speech eudiometry and ABR. It was a case-control study, and 30 healthy volunteers were checked with the matching tools. It was found out that the severity of hearing loss and the graph pattern on PTA varied with the longevity and chronicity of the disease. Abnormal latencies in ABR were noted and found to be associated with high-velocity stimulus. It was pointed out that MS may be diagnosed through detailed audiological evaluation also. A patient presenting with hearing loss with a 'dome-shaped' audiogram and an abnormal gait obviously requires further investigation. Vestibular function tests are not routinely performed in such cases but may be advisable if the patient has any audio-vestibular involvement. Once the diagnosis is made with the help of an MRI, the patient must immediately be referred to the neurology department for further management. Unfortunately the prognosis remains guarded in multiple sclerosis. The essential point to note here is that a simple investigation like a PTA can provide useful clues to the chronicity of this complex clinical condition. Cochlear nerve as well as involvement of more distal pathways of hearing may be responsible for the typical hearing loss in MS. The study concludes that the results of tests like PTA, SDS and ABR can be used as diagnostic aids in MS.

Brown et al. (2006) investigated the hypothesis, if vestibular physical therapy (PT) leads to improved functional outcomes in people with central vestibular dysfunction. The patients were divided into various subgroups including central vestibulopathy, cerebellar dysfunction, stroke, mixed central and peripheral vestibulopathy and post-traumatic central disorders. This study identified significant differences between initial evaluation and discharge in each of the assessment measures for the entire group. Post-hoc tests were performed to determine if there was a significant difference in any of the assessment measures by diagnosis. Central vestibular diagnostic subgroup was shown to affect pre- to post intervention differences in the functional and disability measures, showing statistically significant values.

The final conclusion of the authors was that the patients with central vestibular dysfunctions improved in both subjective and objective measures of balance after physical therapy. But patients with cerebellar dysfunction showed the least improvement. This finding may be of some value to the neurologists.

Vestibular abnormalities in patients with relapsing and remitting multiple sclerosis were investigated by Zeigelboim et al. (2008). This study duly highlights certain pertinence of rehabilitative measures in MS. Thirty patients were evaluated neurologically and through audio-vestibular tests. Vestibular changes were found in 26. Out of which, 25 demonstrated a peripheral cause and only 1 had a central reason. It was also noted that there was a prevalence of bilateral peripheral irritative vestibulopathy, followed by bilateral peripheral deficit vestibulopathy and left peripheral deficit vestibulopathy in that order. The authors commented that specific rehabilitation programmes can be of much assistance in such patients, who suffered with vestibulopathies.

Studies with larger samples are still required and may contribute to the understanding of this pathology. Regrettably many of the patients with MS do not return to us for a follow-up. That leaves us in darkness, though we are confident that they are under the care of physicians who are more versatile and better equipped than us, particularly in dealing with long-term neurological morbidities.

References

Brown KE, Whitney SL, Marchetti GF, Wrisley DM, Furman JM (2006) Physical therapy for central vestibular dysfunction. Arch Phys Med Rehabil 87(1):76–81, 0003–9993

Grayeli AB, Fond C, Kalamarides M, Bouccara D, Cazals-Hatem D, Cyna-Gorse F, Sterkers O (2007) Diagnosis and management of intracochlear schwannomas. Otol Neurotol 28(7):951–957, 1531–7129

Mirz F, Brahe Pedersen C, Fiirgaard B, Lundorf E (2000) Incidence and growth pattern of vestibular schwannomas in a Danish county, 1977–98. Acta Otolaryngol Suppl 543:30–33, 0365–5237

Moffat DA, Jones SEM, Mahendran S, Humphriss R, Baguley DM (2004) Referral patterns in vestibular schwannomas – 10 years on. Clin Otolaryngol Allied Sci 29(5):515–517, 0307–7772

Peyvandi A, Naghibzadeh B, Ahmady Roozbahany N (2010) Neuro-otologic manifestations of multiple sclerosis. Arch Iran Med 13(3):188–192, 1029–2977

Propp JM, McCarthy BJ, Davis FG, Preston-Martin S (2006) Descriptive epidemiology of vestibular schwannomas. Neuro Oncol 8(1):1–11, 1522–8517

Tos M, Charabi S, Thomsen J (1999) Incidence of vestibular schwannomas. Laryngoscope 109(5):736–740, 0023–852X

Ushio M, Iwasaki S, Murofushi T, Sugasawa K, Chhara Y, Fujimoto C, Nakmura M, Yamaguchi T, Yamsoha T (2009) The diagnostic value of vestibular evoked myogenic potential in patients with vestibular schwannoma. Clin Neurophysiol 1206:1149–1153, 1388–24457; 1872–8952

Walton (1977) Understanding multiple sclerosis. In: Robinson I. Rutledge. 1988. Chapter 1. pp 1 (Walton's description of multiple sclerosis 1977: 544)

Zeigelboim BS, Arruda WO, Mangabeira-Albernaz PL, Iorio MCM, Jurkiewicz AL, Martins-Bassetto J, Klagenberg KF (2008) Vestibular findings in relapsing, remitting multiple sclerosis: a study of thirty patients. Int Tinnitus J 14(2):139–145, 0946–5448

General Causes

9

9.1 Cardiovascular Diseases

The general practitioners normally handle most of the non-vestibular cases of vertigo. But sometimes the patient may be referred to an audiology clinic for hearing loss when he mentions about the sudden attack of momentary dizziness, which my therefore require further evaluation.

One of the essential causes of fleeting imbalance could be a cardiovascular condition. Detailed history should therefore be taken particularly for an undiagnosed or uncontrolled hypertension, angina and myocardial infarction, coronary bypass surgery, coils or stents. Some patients may also have other cardiac conditions like bradycardia caused by a defective SA node or a heart block. A patient with Wenckebach phenomenon may present with light-headedness, even dizziness, requiring urgent pacemaker fitting.

A man of 65 presented to us with the complaints of periodic episodes of light-headedness, momentary feeling of shortness of breath and fatigue. After a routine checkup, he was immediately referred to the medical colleagues, who recorded an ECG, which showed a classical picture of Wenckebach phenomenon. He was soon after fitted with a pacemaker with total recovery from light-headedness and fatigue. Timely intervention may have saved him from a serious catastrophe. Referral to a relevant physician must remain an essential component of a fine health delivery system.

Postural hypotension is a fairly common disorder in the elderly population and should be kept in mind as a differential diagnosis. There are some patients who may have been on medications for years without bothering to go back for a review or a checkup. Those medicines may sometimes be either not needed or may perhaps be causing more harm than benefit.

In CVS-triggered dizziness, one must remember that it is the diminished or indeed compromised state of the arterial supply to the brain that is causing the symptoms. Some of the essential causes to remember are as follows: arrhythmias either fast or slow; orthostatic hypotension; hypovolemia as after a haemorrhage; anaemia, a common cause in many developing countries; myocardial ischaemia;

S.H. Zaidi, A. Sinha, *Vertigo*,
DOI 10.1007/978-3-642-36485-3_9, © Springer-Verlag Berlin Heidelberg 2013

structural cardiac or valuable disease; hypoxia; vasovagal syncope; and drug-induced hypotension or dizziness.

The essential thing to remember in CVS disease is that the dizziness is not rotational. It is more like light-headedness, or syncope or presyncope. It is caused by impaired cardiac output leading to decline in the oxygen saturation level of the brain and is usually a passing phase. A state of presyncope is a warning sign to the patient to adopt a posture more suitable to resume the cerebral arterial circulation, hence often enough if the patient sits down from a standing position or lie down just for a short while. If the cerebral circulation badly suffers, he may even collapse on the floor, when the body posture reflexly corrects the head posture facilitating the arterial circulation towards the brain. More severe cases are known to suffer a TIA, even a stroke.

Even in a normal person, the sensation of momentary light-headedness after a heavy meal is a common experience. It is caused by postprandial circulatory changes due to the physiological reasons. In postprandial light-headedness, the circulation is temporarily diverted from the brain and other organs to the digestive system, albeit only temporarily or else it may lead to a state of syncope.

Dizziness caused by cardiac arrhythmias due to inefficient cardiac output may warrant an urgent attention.

Brady-arrhythmias and tachy-arrhythmias can both potentially lead to acute cerebral arterial circulatory deficiency. Syncope may indeed ensue. Adams–Stokes syndrome is one such example to remember. Likewise, in certain electrophysiological conditions of the heart, where the SA node, the AV node or the conducting system is deficient leading to different degrees of heart block, a state of light-headedness may indeed be the first sign of urgent need for attention to the CVS. If neglected, the patient may experience presyncope or syncope. Further delay may eventually lead to complete heart block even cardiac arrest and fatality.

Cardiac muscle may be damaged by a coronary artery disease, which may be the underlying cause of light-headedness and dizziness. Likewise, valvular disease or cardiac myopathies may also lead to vertiginous symptoms.

A cardiologist in the USA explained it explicitly that either you have a plumbing fault or an electrical fault in the heart, i.e. a coronary artery disease or a SA/AV node disease. And both can lead to light-headedness, presyncope or syncope.

Orthostatic hypotension is a known cause of momentary dizziness. It may be drug induced as a patient on cardiac drugs may present with dizziness. Anaemia is also a factor to keep in mind in some situations. As a matter of fact, it is the commonest cause of momentary light-headedness, presyncope and shortness of breath.

9.2　Vertebrobasilar Insufficiency

Vertebral artery arises from the second part of the subclavian artery and has a rather tortuous course, as it traverses the cervical vertebral column only to emerge out at the atlanto-occipital joint, to join the opposite number and enter the skull forming the all important basilar artery. It is the basilar artery that forms the essential posterior supply system for the completion of the Circle of Willis. The later is responsible for supplying the pons, medulla, cerebellum, cerebellopontine angle and beyond.

The commonest causes of vertebrobasilar diseases are embolism, atherosclerotic disease, small (penetrating) artery disease and arterial dissection.

Pathology within the vertebrobasilar system results in either recurrent episodes of transient neurological deficits lasting minutes (vertebrobasilar insufficiency) transient ischaemic attacks (TIA) or indeed cerebrovascular accidents.

It is commonly seen in ageing population though not always so. One of the commonest problems noticed by elderly population is that of imbalance. Jahn et al. (2010) in a study rightly pointed out that gait disturbance is a common problem in the elderly. Limited or reduced mobility markedly impairs quality of life, and associated falls do indeed cause many other allied problems. All clinicians are aware of the fact that comorbidities are common in the elderly. They have duly highlighted several factors responsible for gait disturbances in these patients. Some of them are visual, vestibular, somatosensory, neurodegenerative such as cortical, extrapyramidal motor, cerebellar toxic such as caused by drugs and anxiety for primary or concerning falls.

Up to 25 % of patients with VBD show up in the clinic with an attack of vertigo. Many others may have more intense symptoms. Since anterior inferior cerebellar and the posterior inferior cerebellar arteries, both branches of the basilar artery, supply the central controls for maintenance of balance, namely, the pons, medulla and the cerebellum, numerous syndromes have been identified to result following a severe insult to this vascular system resulting in ischaemic changes, even an infarct. One well-known syndrome is called the lateral medullary syndrome of Wallenberg. It results from ischaemia of the posterior inferior cerebellar artery.

Some of these patients may present with vertigo, tinnitus and hearing impairment, while others may come to our ENT clinics for facial pain and weakness, ataxia, Horner's syndrome, hoarseness caused by laryngeal nerve paralysis or dysphasia caused by pharyngo-laryngeal involvement. Videofluoroscopy and contrast medium video-pharyngo-laryngography are invaluable tools, in establishing the diagnosis. MRI is of course mandatory in all these patients. Many would also require MRA (magnetic resonance angiography) to identify the vasculature of the affected territory. CT imaging has almost taken over many conventional stress tests in the CVS diseases in major centres in the USA and some centres in the UK. Therefore, a specialist trained in cardiac imaging may be of immense values in some of these patients, who obviously have CVS disease underlying all the effects arising there from. A Doppler study is of immense value in these patients.

Vestibular-evoked myogenic potentials have taken up the task of early and prompt diagnosis and monitoring the progress of the disease, in many difficult cases. This tool is the subject of study in many centres. Deftereos et al. (2006) evaluated the use of vestibular-evoked myogenic potentials (VEMPs) in the assessment of neural function, following medullary lesions in a middle-aged man with typical features of right lateral medullary (Wallenberg) syndrome. MRI and three successive neurophysiological investigations, which included VEMPs, brainstem auditory-evoked responses (BAERs) and the blink reflex, were carried out.

Following the investigation, it was noted that VEMPs amplitude progressively increased, parallel to the improvement of vestibular symptoms. The blink reflex evolved differently, while BAERs were not affected. As the three evoked responses are mediated by separate neural circuits, they provide information on different aspects of brainstem function. Thus, VEMPs seemed to be a useful tool, which complements the existing methods employed in the assessment of brainstem lesions.

Prognosis depends upon the severity of ischaemia. Acute cases of VBA have poor prognosis, while the mild to moderated degree of ischaemia may allow the development of collaterals and recanalisation with some improvement. Some symptoms like hoarseness, repeated chest infections due to spill over and dysphagia may require rehabilitative measures on long-term basis. Such patients greatly benefit with rehabilitation therapy. The role of our team in the speech and language therapy as well as the rehabilitation team deserves many accolades in the management of these patients with amazing results.

9.3   Noise

Noise is an ancient cause of damage to human health. Ancient Greece was quiet and sedate. People had time to think and reflect, thus gifting the mankind with such sophists as Pythagoras and Protagoras, before the emergence of all-time greats like Socrates, Plato and Aristotle. The world still reaps harvest of the seeds of wisdom sowed by those men of intellect three millennia ago.

Then came the Romans in their mighty chariots and war wagons and destroyed the peace, quiet and intellectual growth. The world had discovered wheel, war machinery and noise. Peace of the ancient lands of thinkers and philosophers was trampled under the hooves of angry horses and other ferocious beasts, and the world lost its brain to brawn.

Industrialisation of Europe brought in great economic revolution, at the cost of peace of mind. The world realised the loss after a few centuries and as mentioned here under, some measures were taken.

'Noise has always been an important environmental problem for man. In industry, machinery emits high noise levels and amusement centre and pleasure vehicles distract leisure time relaxation', thus wrote Richard Helmer (1999).

Since 1980, the WHO has been taking active interest in the problems posed by noise. They held several meetings on the subject in 1995; a preliminary publication of the Karolinska Institute, Stockholm, appeared on behalf of the WHO. An international team of experts was then chosen to develop the principles for the world to apply in their territories. The group held several meeting and finally published a document for global application called the Guidelines for Community Noise. It was published in 1999 (Helmer 1999; Berglund et al. 1995).

It duly highlights many adverse effects of noise on human health. Eastern Mediterranean Region of WHO (EMRO) was represented by Zaidi (1989a), who collected a vast amount of epidemiological and statistical data from several countries belonging to the EMRO region. It is a part of the said document.

NIHL of course is a major problem which may be accompanied by tinnitus. The higher frequencies, i.e. 3,000–6,000 Hz, are predominantly affected. Interference with speech and communication, disturbance of rest and sleep; psychological trauma and annoyance etc are some other note able effects.

Noise can affect the vestibular system, a fact known to us since a long time. At the turn of the nineteenth century, Urbantschitsch was able to demonstrate and document nystagmus in response to auditory stimuli (1989) (Oosterveld WJ). The famous physician Tullio showed in the 1930s that exposure to noise in one ear can produce vertiginous symptoms, including an observable nystagmus. This is known as the Tullio phenomenon. The interesting thing about the Tullio phenomenon is that it does not occur on auditory stimulation of both ears due to the fact that the reflexes equalise each other, as was demonstrated by Von Bekesy in 1935.

Experience has taught us that in many countries, the life is mainly outdoors. The noise pollution makes day-to-day life simply unbearable, and many patients exposed to higher levels of noise during day and night have experienced oscillopsia, even dizziness on many occasions. The main sources of noise pollution were identified in several studies conducted by many workers. One such study exposed that leq, 8 h values in the metropolis of Karachi, valued at 80–85 dBA on a normal working day. During the peak rush hours at notoriously busy intersection in Karachi called the Tibet centre, the noise level peaked at 140 dBA at around 5 pm, when the home commuters hit the roads on cars, buses, rickshaws and motorcycles and simply walking Zaidi (1989b).

A study conducted by the same workers on a day of public transporters strike recorded on the identical places with same variables ion terms of technique, distance from the source, recording methods, etc. revealed that the noise level was significantly low dropping from an average of 90 dB to 70 dBA (Zaidi 1990) proving the point that the major source of noise pollution in urban large metropolises like Karachi is the public transport like the buses, rickshaws, trucks and lorries.

In fact, it was identified that the rickshaw can generate a noise level of 110–120 dB (Zaidi 1997; Shams 1997); these tiny but noisy vehicles in Karachi run without the silencers duly removed to save on the cost of diesel. A similar vehicle used in Bangkok called the Tuk Tuk generates much lower noise levels as they run with the silencers duly fitted.

During the volatile days of random firing and bomb blasts, it was a the common experience to see the patients presenting with ruptured ear drums, cochlear concussion, tinnitus oscillopsia, vertigo, syncope, fainting, chronic headaches, fatigue, irritation and suicidal tendencies. Matters are considerably worse now in many parts of the world.

The problem was once duly highlighted in a television drama when an expatriate returning home after several years of sojourn in the UK found himself living next to a small factory illegally established in a residential area. The hammering never stopped during the night or day. The man became so disturbed with insomnia, fatigue, tinnitus and dizziness that after pleading many times to the factory owner to control the noise at least during the night, and having failed to do so, bought a firearm and shot the factory owner dead before surrendering himself to law.

Nowadays, many major cities like London, New York and Moscow have seen worst from of terrorism; surely fresh studies would confirm that noise is a major contributor to the burden of disease on human health. More recently, the public uprising and revolutions across the Arab world, called the Arab Spring as witnessed in Tunis, Cairo, Sanaa, Tripoli, Benghazi, etc., have once again highlighted the impact of noise on generated by bombs, gunfire and explosions, on human health.

Noise does not have only its auditory effect to remember but other impacts also. It is nearly always accompanied with vibration and a shaking effect. Of course it is dependent on the physical intensity, pitch and frequency, but a man who works on a noisy machinery does not complain of experiencing only the effect of noise exposure, which has now considerably controlled with noise defenders, etc., but the vibration that the machine produces that actually shakes the workers' body as if he is sitting in a fast-moving vehicle travelling on a bumpy road. The impact of vibration on the human organs is still an underinvestigated subject. It can bring about imbalance due to the low grade but constant shaking and moving state of the labyrinthine fluids and the delicate hair cellars, the otoconia, the cupola, the utricle and the saccule. All these structures are very, very fine in texture and rest upon each other in an extremely fragile relationship. A violent shake as experienced after a blast or a constant, low-graded vibration produced by the noisy machinery can both bring about damage to the delicate neuroepithelial structures, which are usually irreparable.

Vestibular damage, however, on exposure to noise is relatively less common, perhaps less reported, than the cochlear damage. Temporary threshold shift (TTS) as well as permanent threshold shifts (PTS) are well-documented effects of noise on human ears. Imbalance, tinnitus, headaches and fatigue are fairly common but relatively less-documented sequelae of exposure to loud noise. Permanent loss is particularly prominent 4,000 and 6,000 Hz, which is considered to be almost a diagnostic feature of noise-induced hearing loss (Fig. 9.1).

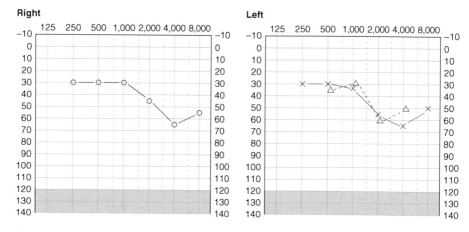

Fig. 9.1 This pure tone audiogram shows bilateral sensorineural hearing loss in a patient with a history of noise exposure for many years, without using ear defenders. The loss is mild to moderate (30–40 dB) in the lower frequencies and moderate to severe (40–70 dB) in intensity in higher frequencies. The dip at 4,000 cpc is almost pathognomonic of noise-induced hearing loss (NIHL). The hearing level in the right ear is recorded in *red colour* and in *blue colour* in the left ear

Glottal and colleagues (2001) reported their study which was conducted in 2001 on 258 military subjects who had been heavily exposed to noise. They found that vestibular damage caused by intense noise exposure might be expressed clinically in subjects with asymmetrical hearing loss. They noted that there was a strong correlation between the subjects' complaints and the results of the VFT. They also noted that there was no correlation between the severity of the hearing loss and the vestibular symptoms. Therefore, they inferred from their study that thus exposed to intense noise may have some proof of vestibular damage only when the hearing loss was asymmetrical. They also noted that whenever hearing loss was symmetrical, an equal damage to the vestibular systems of both ears is most probably responsible for the absence of abnormal findings on the vestibular function tests. This study bears marked importance upon the medicolegal implications of those exposed to intense noise.

Another study was published by Oosterveld (1989) in which extensive vestibular investigation was carried out in 29 subjects exposed to loud noise. It reported positive presence of spontaneous nystagmus in 18 subjects and positional nystagmus exceeding a velocity of the slow phase of 5° in 3 or more subjects. In another 17 subjects, a cervical nystagmus could be elicited, while a nystagmus preponderance of more than 20 % in the rotation test was found in 7 subjects. A difference in excitability between the labyrinths of more than 20 % was shown by 7 subjects. None showed vestibular pathology per se. All subjects showed pathology in one or more of the hearing tests. Hearing loss itself could not affect work capability, the authors opined, but a vestibular disorder may well do so. In consequence, noise-exposed persons could be disabled on account of vertigo or imbalance. The authors noted that it is an important and perhaps neglected aspect of noise-induced hearing damage.

In 1997, a study demonstrated that noise can indeed cause potential damage to the vestibular system. Aantaa et al. (1982) investigated and reported findings in 49 male workers, who had been working in extremely noisy environment and vibration between 6 months and 10 years. Spontaneous nystagmus could be seen as indeed hypofunctioning on calorimetry or pathology in rotational test in 44.9 % of the subjects. It was believed that the lesion may have involved the peripheral vestibular organ as a consequence of low-frequency vibration.

Shupak et al. (1977) evaluated the vestibular function in a group of cohorts with documented NIHL. They employed ENG and the Smooth Harmonic Acceleration (SHA) test in their investigative research. This study duly highlighted a symmetrical centrally compensated decrease in the vestibular end-organ response which was associated with the symmetrical hearing loss measured in the study group.

Statistically significant correlation was found between the average hearing loss, the decrease in the average vestibulo-ocular reflex gain ($p = 0.01$) and ENG caloric lateralisation ($p = 0.02$).

Their results imply subclinical well-compensated malfunction of the vestibular system associated with NIH. It is possible that a single mechanism may exist for both cochlear and vestibular noise-induced hearing loss. It requires further evaluation and more studies, as currently the literature is deficient on this subject. One fears that the nuisance of noise and vibration leading to vestibular damage may be quite significant, particularly in factory workers, where huge machines make very, very loud noise along with massive vibration. Obviously a correlation between cochlear and vestibular loss following noise exposure exists, as was duly highlighted by this study.

Scherer and Schubert (1994) did a study summarising the findings and effects of blasts, reviewing relevant patient's characteristics and sensor motor deficits associated with blast injuries and suggesting clinical best practices for the rehabilitation of such patients suffering with dizziness. They duly highlighted the importance of dizziness as a common complaint in soldiers returning from wars in Afghanistan and Iraq following exposure to blasts. Some of these soldiers complained of vertigo, gaze instability, motion intolerance and symptoms of peripheral vestibular pathology.

One of the investigations gaining popularity is the vestibular-evoked myogenic potential vestibulometry. Kumar and colleagues (2009) looked at it in 30 patients (55 ears) with NIHL. VEMP was recorded at 99 dBnhl using HIS instrument. The results were quite interesting as they showed that as the average pure tone threshold increased, the latencies of VEMPs were also prolonged and peak-to-peak amplitude was reduced in subjects with NIHL. The conclusion of their study was that the possibility of vestibular dysfunction especially the saccular pathways is high in NIHL. They recommended that VEMP being a noninvasive procedure may be employed in such individuals.

The exact mechanism of vestibular damage in noise exposure remains to be established. Kacker and Hinchcliffe proposed the possibility of the excessive vibration of the membranous labyrinth as a possible cause, as mentioned by Oosterveld in his article (Kumar et al. 2010). He also quotes McCabe and Lawrence, who reported in 1958 that the damaging effect of noise upon the vestibular organ was restricted to the cochlea and macula but the semicircular canals and the utricle did not get affected. The basal turn of cochlea and the saccule seem to bear the maximum brunt of noise-induced trauma. It could well be due to the fact that embryologically the semicircular canals develop from the utricle and the cochlear duct developed from the saccule.

Can noise lead to the development of an acoustic neuroma? Preston et al. (1989) noticed a co-relationship between occupations involving exposure to extremely loud noise and an acoustic neuroma.

Propp et al. (2006) felt that men working in loud noise environment for 20 or more years were twice as more likely to develop these tumours than individuals who were not exposed to such a noise.

These workers also mention that cellular phones causing brain tumours is currently under a study by the International Agency for Research on Cancer involving as a study of acoustic neuromas and other brain tumours. It is hypothesised that two lines of evidence support this work. The vestibular schwannomas are situated within the direct line of the radio-frequency exposure near the ear and that could be one possibility. The second possibility could be that in a cohort study of persons exposed to high-dose radiation, the relative risks associated with developing nerve sheath tumours were very high.

Obviously one waits to hear the final results of the research currently under way.

Suffice it to say that noise has enormous impact on human life. It does not remain confined to the hearing loss only, which is permanent at 4 K, but can also affect the balance, sleep, psyche, CVS and overall health of a human being. Protection from noise exposure is the best way to save one from its many hazards.

Noise protection gear is mandatory in all noisy work place in the UK and elsewhere. But many a patient presenting for hearing assessment in our clinics often say that they avoid wearing the ear defenders, because it isolates them from the environment, making them vulnerable to physical accidents. They often complain of tinnitus and sometimes chronic imbalance.

9.4 Miscellaneous Causes of Vertigo

Numerous causes may be included in this group. Iatrogenic is an example to remember.

It is a common observation that as simple a procedure as springing of the ear may lead to momentary dizziness, even an intense bout of vertigo. All of us who have been in practice for some time have encountered an odd case of the vasovagal stimulation leading to presyncope, even collapse.

That is why it is a traditional teaching that before springing, one must check the temperature of the water or saline used for the purpose. It should be at the room temperature. If it is too cold or too warm, it will stimulate the labyrinth, as the temperature in the ear canal would induce convention currents that will be conducted through the tympanic membrane into the middle ear changing the middle ear temperature, leading to transmission of the impulse to the inner ear. It may lead to a passing phase of minor imbalance but may sometimes lead to intense and volatile vertigo, even vasovagal symptoms such as nausea, sickness, sweating, pallor, presyncope or outright momentary fall. The vasovagal stimulus is brought about by irritation of the auricular branch of vagus nerve, which supplies a tiny component of the eardrum with sensory innervation. One must remember the golden rule while springing. The syringe should be pointed upwards, backwards and laterally, i.e. towards the upper pole of pinna. It would thus avoid any traumatic perforation of the eardrum, as indeed diminish the chances of direct stimulation of the tympanic membrane, resulting in a caloric effect on the labyrinth.

A similar caloric response may be seen in an odd healthy ear, during a microsuction, but more commonly in mastoid cavities, which often return to us for an aural toilet. It may sometimes precipitate vertigo, due to stimulation of the labyrinthine capsule, a caloric brought about by the stimulation of the labyrinth. Simple measures like allowing the patient to rest a few moments on a couch with eyes closed would soon ease the symptoms. Sometimes, however, the procedure may have to be abandoned. A positive evidence of the stimulation of the labyrinthine capsule in mastoid cavity, during an aural toilet, is a horizontal nystagmus which beats contralaterally and is fatigue able.

Another common cause to be mentioned here is the role of certain drugs prescribed by a physician. It could either be an idiosyncrasy or an allergic reaction to a particular drug, or simply incorrect dosage of a medicine, or indeed an excessive quantity, perhaps inadvertently ingested by the patient. Many cardiac drugs are known to potentate imbalance, and the patient has just to inform the family physician, who may either withhold or adjust the dosage. Likewise antidiabetic drugs may lead to iatrogenic hypo- or hyperglycaemia causing imbalance.

Numerous other miscellaneous causes of vertigo have been mentioned in the literature. One such unusual condition described by Kulahi et al. (2005) is that of Behcet's syndrome.

This study was carried out to determine the characteristics and incidence of hearing loss and vestibular disturbance in Behcet's syndrome with a large number of patients. Sixty-two patients with Behcet's syndrome were included in this study; 62 healthy normal control subjects (38 male and 24 female) were included. Patient and control groups were questioned about any history of audio-vestibular disturbance and underwent physical and ENT examination and the following audiological tests: pure tone audiometric test (0.25, 0.5, 1, 2, 4 and 6 kHz), tympanogram, speech discrimination, short increment sensitivity index, tone-decay test and auditory brainstem response. Vestibular system was evaluated by a VNG and calorimetry. MRI of patients who had vestibular disturbances were requested to examine the central nervous system. Both the patient and the control groups were tested with the HLA-B51 antigen. Pure tone audiogram showed sensorineural hearing loss (25 dB hearing level in at least two frequencies) in 20 of the 62 (32 %) Behcet's patients, while the control group were normal. There was a hearing loss involving high frequencies in the audiograms of Behcet's patients with hearing disturbances. The recruitment investigation tests and auditory brainstem response confirmed cochlear involvement in all 20 patients. Caloric stimulation tests revealed a normal vestibular function in all patient and control group. In electronystagmography, 21 (34 %) patients had hypo- or hypermetric saccades and smooth pursuit tests showing that 4 (6 %) patients had pathological changes while the control group was normal. HLA-B51 antigen was found positive in 15 of 20 Behcet's patient with hearing loss.

The study concluded that (1) the hearing and vestibular disturbances in Behcet's syndrome was more prevalent than previously recognised, (2) hearing loss in high frequencies in Behcet's patients is an indicator of cochlear involvement in this disease, (3) there is a higher prevalence of central vestibular syndrome in Behcet's patients than it was thought before and (4) HLA-B51 antigen may be able to be a prognostic factor for sensorineural hearing loss in Behcet's patients.

References

Aantaa E, Virolaien E, Karskela V (1977) Permanent effects of low frequency vibration on the vestibular system. Acta Otolaryngol 83(5–6):470–474

Berglund B, Lindvall T, Scwella D (eds) (1995) Guidelines for community noise. WHO, Geneva

Deftereos SN, Panagopoulos G, Gryllia M, Georgonikou D, Polyzoi M (2006) Neurophysiological monitoring of brainstem function in a patient with Wallenberg syndrome, using vestibular evoked myogenic potentials. Neurol Neurophysiol Neurosci 3:1233–1266

Golz A, Westerman ST, Westerman LM et al (2001) The effects of noise on the vestibular system. Am J Otolaryngol 22(3):190–196

Helmer R (1999) Protection of the human environment, in the foreword of the globally acknowledged document called 'guidelines for community noise' published by the WHO in 1999.

Jahn K, Zwergal A, Schniepp R (2010) Gait disturbances in old age. Dtch Arztebl Int 107(17):306–316, 0012–1207

Kulahli I, Balci K, Koseoglu E, Yuce I, Cagli S, Senturk M (2005) Audio-vestibular disturbances in Behcet's patients: report of 62 cases. Hear Res 203(1–2):28–31, 0378–5955; 0378–5955

Kumar K, Vivarthini CJ, Bhat JS (2010) Vestibular evoked myogenic potential in NIHL. Noise Health 12(48):191–194, 1463–1741

Oosterveld WJ, Polman AR, Schoneheyt J (1982) Vestibular implications of NIHL. Br J Audiol 16(4):227–232

Preston-Martin S, Thomas DC, Wright WE, Henderson BE (1989) Noise trauma in aetiology of acoustic neuromas in men in Los Angeles county, 1978–1985. Br J Caner 59:783–786

Propp JM et al (2006) Descriptive epidemiology of vestibular schwannomas. Neuro Oncol 8(1):1–11

Scherer MR, Schubert MC (2009) Traumatic brain injury and vestibular pathology as a co morbidity after blast exposure. Phys Ther 89(9):980–992, 0031–9023; 1538–6724

Shams A (1997) The hazards of noise pollution. Daily Dawn. 10 Sept 1997

Shupak A, Bar-E El E, Podoshin L, Spitzer O, Gordon CR et al (1994) Vestibular findings associated with chronic NIHL. Acta Otolaryngol 114(6):579–585

Zaidi SH (1989a) Noise levels and sources of noise pollution in Karachi. J Pak Med Assoc 39:62–65

Zaidi S (1989b) How safe is noise? Pak J Otolaryngol 30:60–61

Zaidi S (1990) Noise levels in Karachi, on a transporters strikes day. J Pak Med Assoc 40:299–300

Zaidi S (1997) Noise induced hearing loss. Hear Int 6(3):12–13

Paediatric Clinical Conditions

10

10.1 Vertigo in Children

The literature is relatively deficient on the subject of paediatric vertigo. As a matter of fact, you need to have a special interest in this field to indulge into this problem at length.

Generally it is believed that vertigo is a rare clinical condition in children showing its prevalence to be under 1 % (Fried 1980; Eviatar and Eviatar 1977).

A population-based study was carried out in Scotland by Abu-Arafeh and Russell (1995), which is a genuine reflection on the prevalence of vertigo in the school going children. It documented that 18 % of 5–15-year-olds would have had at least one attack of vertigo during the past 1 year and 5 % more than three attacks. Furthermore, it discusses the salient contributors to the aetiopathogenesis of vertigo on this age group, duly highlighting such contributors as migraine, positional vertigo and vestibulopathies.

Vertigo may present itself in many forms in children. The younger the child, the more challenging the diagnostic dilemma and its management would be. It may present as an acute attack of vertigo which may be easy to pick up or a chronic state of imbalance, which the child may not be able to describe precisely. Sometimes, besides the classical symptoms of perception of movement of objects, the child may complain of nausea, vomiting and abdominal discomfort or develop ataxia. Headache, loss of appetite, irritability, lassitude, diplopia, hearing loss, earache, hyperacusis, phonophobia or frank otorrhoea may be some other presentations.

Headache is a common problem in children. It can be caused by numerous underlying conditions, such as an error of refraction, anaemia, viral infections and febrile illnesses. If a child complains of headache followed by vertigo, nausea and sickness, sometimes then one must suspect migrainous vertigo as a possibility.

Some of these children may have underlying ocular problems like strabismus or simply an error of refraction, which obviously needs referral to an optometrist or an ophthalmologist.

Vertigo in children may be the result of impaired functioning of the three sensory components involved in the maintenance of balance. They are the vestibular, the

S.H. Zaidi, A. Sinha, *Vertigo*,
DOI 10.1007/978-3-642-36485-3_10, © Springer-Verlag Berlin Heidelberg 2013

ocular and the central nervous system. All of them may be affected with a disease to result in imbalance.

Vertigo in children may be an acute state or a chronic relapsing recurrent dizziness. A child may show his vertigo in the form of a tendency to fall or being noble to walk straight without bumping into objects. Ataxia, loss of appetite, nausea and sickness may be symptoms and signs in a child.

Case Report

P was born in late 1990s and was referred to the vestibular lab at City and Sandwell hospital for further investigation. He was seen in the lab in 2011 when he said that he had been experiencing rotatory vertigo for the last 3–4 years. These spells lasted a few minutes, but he felt disorientated and drained for approximately 30 min afterwards. He said that the people around sounded as if they were mumbling rather than talking just before an attack. His mum said that he had a vacant look in his eyes and increased rebate of breathing during the episode. His heart rate also went up, the mum said. During an attack of dizziness, P felt better if he held onto his mother and if he concentrated on something. Spells appeared to be spontaneous but happened more whenever he was in a crowd. He also felt flashing lights could provoke an attack. He therefore wore tinted glasses, as he was photosensitive. P felt nervous on leaving his house. There was no history of nausea, vomiting, falls and loss of consciousness. He felt constant dizzy between the attacks, though lately felt well in between the attacks.

P first experienced a dizzy spell at the time when he had a febrile illness and had become disoriented and incoherent. He had also noted that his vision had gone blank and he failed to concentrate. The mums said that he was a late walker (18 months) and slow to start reading, though he picked up in due course.

He had no hearing loss, or tinnitus is indeed an ear disease per se. His GP thought it could be an epileptic form. P therefore had an MRI, ECG and EEG, which were all reported to be normal.

His otoscopy was normal. The tympanometry showed normal middle ear pressure bilaterally, and the PTA was also normal.

On functional testing P was able to maintain his balance with reduced visual and proprioceptive inputs. Oculomotor testing using VNG revealed no spontaneous, gaze-evoked or rebound nystagmus. Testing of random saccades and smooth pursuit revealed no abnormalities. Dix–Hallpike test was not indicated in his history. Water calorimetry was not undertaken as he was very anxious even during tympanometry. Rotatory chair, head shaking, and head thrust testing did not indicate any large asymmetry in vestibular function. Nijmegen questionnaire results did not indicate hyperventilation syndrome.

It was therefore inferred that P did not have a central or peripheral vestibular pathology, though calorimetry would have been ideal. He was finally referred for relaxation therapy.

P attended the clinic, when mum told the attending doctor that within a few weeks of relaxation therapy, P has shown remarkable improvement and is neither dizzy nor stressed out. In fact, he had now started venturing out of the house with confidence. P was given a follow-up appointment in 3 months to monitor his progress.

Headache in a child may not be an ordinary headache, as it could well be either a migraine or migrainous equivalent, which is commoner than duly appreciated by most clinicians. Migrainous equivalents are common enough, but often overshadowed by errors of refraction, stays us or other ophthalmological manifestations. They must be checked by a paediatric ophthalmologist. Besides, there may be certain trigger factors such as bullying at school, stress at school due to academic- or teacher-related issues, psychological factors, lack of sleep and certain food elements.

Early-age episodes of migraine equivalent vertigo, not responding to simple preventive and therapeutic measures, and frequently repeated attacks, almost developing a pattern such as monthly or fortnightly episodes, with uncontrollable nausea, and familial history of migraine should not be taken lightly.

Paediatric consultation may be necessary in some others cases where recurrent migrainous attacks with associated symptoms of vertigo may make a child's life miserable. A condition called episodic ataxia type II, which is genetic and familial in nature, may need to be excluded. Acetazolamide can avert the crisis and is in fact a diagnostic tool as well. L-leucine is also a useful therapy and should be tried first as acetazolamide may result in renal lithiasis over prolonged use (Niemensivu et al. 2006). This study included over a thousand children, who were sent a questionnaire on their dizzy symptoms. In response, 89 % or a carer completed a simple screening questionnaire. Eight percent had experienced vertigo, and 23 % of these suffered very severe vertigo that it prevented their present activity. In 30 % of the children, no reason could be identified. But 69 % could name a provocative factor. Obviously balance disorders are not quite so uncommon in children, simply less diagnosed.

A common cause of vertigo in children is a head injury, as it may account for about 10 % of all cases of vertigo (Wiener-Vacher 2008). With the strict rules of wearing protective head gear while cycling, climbing up the walls, etc. in theme parks, its incidence has dramatically reduced. Accidents, however, do happen, and head injury may result in a fracture of the temporal bone. It has been discussed elsewhere in some detail, but suffice it to say that a child with a history of fall or accident deserves a thorough clinical and often radiological examination. Temporal bone may fracture longitudinally or transversely. Depending on the location of the fracture line, the inner ear may or may not escape. CSF rhinorrhoea is a definite sign in such situations to warrant an ENT examination, a CT scan and perhaps an opinion of a neurosurgeon. Sometimes tiny fracture may be invisible in children and can be easily missed out and may present as a case of chronic intractable headache and signs of realised intracranial pressure or, worse, meningitis. Radiology plays a significant role, despite its limitation in delineating a paediatric fracture line. It may show an air bubble in the labyrinth, indicating the communication between the inner and middle ear. It is a transitory sign, disappearing in less than 8 days, or indeed the development of a labyrinthine fistula requiring urgent surgical repair (Wiener-Vacher 2008).

Dilated vestibular aqueduct syndrome is a rare congenital condition, seen in the children in paediatric audiological clinics. It is very unusual in presentation, and unless one is cognizant of its existence, it may indeed be missed out. Typically the child has fluctuating hearing loss with repeated bouts of vertigo. The hearing loss is sensorineural and progressive in nature, but more importantly, it is the state of vertigo that not only shakes up the child's confidence but is equally worrying for the parents. The clinical examination of the ear is satisfactory, but an MRI/CT scan is mandatory. It should confirm the diagnosis. CT scan in a child is a lot easier as it is fast and may not require sedation, while MRI would necessitate sedation. The treatment is conservative. A family has recently been diagnosed in our clinics, to have dilated vestibular aqueduct syndrome. Further studies are under way to define the underlying factors including genetics and other possible factors.

Case Report

P, 12 years of age, was investigated in our vestibular lab in April 2007 for his balance problem. His history of dizziness went back 5 years. His mum said that following a viral or a febrile ear infection, P felt spinning sensation accompanied with nausea. A year and a half after the onset of these episodes, the pattern changed so that the dizziness always preceded the illness. The episodes had remained like this since then. Typically he felt dizzy for an hour and could resume normal daily activities soon after. There had been several such episodes which left P debilitated for days.

In the recent past he had two significant episodes. In December 2005, P had a bout of cold or flu with marked dizziness which lasted for days. It took him 4 weeks to fully recover. In August 2006, P had true rotatory vertigo which lasted 3 days. His hearing deteriorated in his left ear at the time of the onset of dizziness but returned to pre-dizziness level gradually after the attack. The only thing that provoked his dizziness was loud sounds, such as a teacher shouting through his radio aid at school. P walked at 18 months of age. His mum thought that he was slow to start, though had no difficulties in walking.

P wears hearing aids in both ears, and mum thought that his hearing fluctuated though he had not experienced any significant deterioration in his hearing. His hearing was never affected adversely whenever he was dizzy. He sometimes had a unilateral tinnitus, which was not associated with his dizziness, though he could not figure out which ear was affected with tinnitus.

On otoscopy and tympanometry, nothing significant was noted. PTA showed bilateral severe mixed hearing loss. Small changes were noted in his hearing level compared with previous tests, suggesting some degree of fluctuation. P had an MRI scan done previously at a children's hospital. Our vestibular lab performed screening tests for his peripheral vestibular function. He struggled to maintain his balance with visual and proprioceptive inputs reduced, although he did succeed on his third attempt. On examination of his post-rotational nystagmus, no significant nystagmus was observed following rotation to the left, which might indicate a significant asymmetry in vestibular function.

P's history and the test results were found to be consistent with asymmetric vestibular functions. Calorimetry was therefore scheduled for a later date.

A CT scan was requested by the clinician to establish the diagnosis, which confirmed that P indeed had dilated vestibular aqueduct.

Benign paroxysmal positional vertigo is perhaps the second commonest cause of vertigo in children, particularly in infants affecting approximately 20 % of all cases (Wiener-Vacher 2008). The episodes are infrequent and temporarily debilitating. One must take a comprehensive history to eliminate other possible causes before labelling it as BPPV. Vestibular test as mentioned in this book may be employed, particularly a ROTO test, but imaging should be avoided as we do in most paediatric conditions, so as to avoid a general anaesthesia, unless absolutely indispensable.

Vestibular neuronitis is said to affect about 5 % of the children (Wiener-Vacher 2008). It may be difficult to diagnose easily, but a history of an acute episode of vertigo without a concomitant history of otitis media which may lead to a bacterial labyrinthitis is always helpful. A positive Unterberger's test and a positive Romberg's test with tendency to fall ipsilaterally will almost confirm the vestibular involvement.

Berrettini et al. (2005) carried out a study to analyse the clinical, audiological, radiological and genetic features in 17 patients affected with large vestibular aqueduct syndrome (LVAS). They employed very sophisticated equipment in their investigation. High-resolution magnetic resonance imaging of the inner ear, with 3-dimensional reconstructions of the labyrinth and high-resolution spiral computed tomography of the temporal bone, were employed as the diagnostic tools. Some older patients were submitted to a complete audiological evaluation, a thyroid function test, an ultrasound and a molecular study of the PDS gene.

This study showed that the clinical presentation of LVAS was very variable in those patients. The enlarged vestibular aqueduct syndrome was found to be bilateral in 15 cases and unilateral in others. It was the only malformation of the labyrinth in

12 patients, whereas it was associated with other inner ear anomalies in the other 5. The hearing loss was very variable in degree (from mild to profound), age at onset and progression. Moreover, ten children also had Pendred's syndrome (PS), three by distal renal tubular acidosis associated with large vestibular aqueduct, whereas in other three patients the large vestibular aqueduct was non-syndromal. The authors also identified mutations in the PDS gene in five of ten patients with this syndrome. The conclusion of the study was that their data underscored the frequent role of the large vestibular aqueduct syndrome in the pathogenesis of sensorineural hearing loss and the overall wide variability in its audiological features. It also highlighted that LVAS is often part of some syndromal diseases, such as Pendred's, which is often misdiagnosed because of the varying degree of thyroid symptoms. This study also underscored the possible role of hydro-electrolyte and acid–base imbalance or endolymphatic fluid disorders in the pathogenesis of enlarged vestibular aqueduct syndrome.

There is an anatomical variation in this clinical condition leading to vertiginous attacks in children. Unless one is aware of it, one may not fully understand its implications.

Studies have been carried out to evaluate the anatomical and functional parameters in large vestibular aqueduct syndrome. LVAS evident on MRI and correlated with the clinical data was investigated for endolymphatic evidence of incomplete cochlear positioning and sac heterogeneity. The final outcome was a clear message to a clinician that anatomical variations can be easily diagnosed through an MRI, which is an invaluable tool in the diagnosis of dilated vestibular aqueduct syndrome.

An important indeed essential investigation of course is the vestibulometry, which is always challenging in children. An office procedure was described by Maki-Torkko and Magnusson (2005) which may make the life of a clinician a little bit easier.

They mention that since coexisting vestibular and cochlear lesions are of etiological importance, evaluation of children with congenital or early acquired hearing impairment should include vestibular assessment. Discussing the merits and limitations of various vestibular diagnostic tests, they mentioned that the rotation test requires specific equipment and allows confirmation of bilateral vestibular impairment only, while the head thrust test allows assessment of one ear at a time. Furthermore, it detects more pronounced caloric side differences and needs no equipment. They reported a consecutive series of children with profound sensorineural hearing impairment investigated at a tertiary hospital unit. Essential milestones like the age at taking first step without help, the results of imaging of the temporal bones and vestibular tests were collected retrospectively from the records. The children were 12–90 months old at the time they attended both a rotation and an impulse test. All 14 children cooperated in the impulse test, and 12 completed the vestibular rotation test successfully. They went on to claim in the study that 3 out of 14 children tested were subsequently proved to have a bilateral pathological vestibulo-ocular reflex, duly confirmed both in the rotation test and the impulse test. Maki-Torkko and Magnusson (2005) also noted that coexisting vestibular and cochlear lesions are of etiological importance. Therefore, they believe that evaluation of children with congenital or early acquired hearing impairment should include vestibular assessment. They opined that a rotation test requires specific equipment and allows only detection of bilateral vestibular impairment. An impulse or head thrust test allows assessment of one ear at a time and detects more pronounced caloric side differences. Besides, it needs no equipment. They reported a series of children with profound sensorineural hearing impairment investigated at a tertiary hospital unit. They claim that their results showed that both the rotation test and the vestibular impulse test can be successfully performed on small children as an outpatient procedure.

Suffice it to say that it is a simple and useful study which shows that simple measures like the head impulse test can be extremely useful tools in the diagnosis of vertigo. A rotational chair test is still a time-consuming and equipment needing test, but the former is simple, logistically easy and should be employed more routinely than it is, at present.

For an inexplicable reason, dizziness caused by vestibular disorders is considered to be uncommon in children. Partly it is due to their difficulty in expressing their feelings adequately enough. For instance, a child may complain of headache and not dizziness only to be suspected by the mum if the child throws up.

Many causes have been identified to cause vertigo in children, including the Meniere's disease. It has been described as 100 times less frequent than in adults (Worden and Blevins 2007). It was investigated by Aust and Novotny (2005) as a possible diagnosis in a study. They noted that vertigo in children is less frequent than in adults, and examiners of patients showing these symptoms must rely on parents or relatives' observations and statements. This is absolutely true. Besides, the balance disorders can be caused by hereditary malabsorption syndromes or lesions in the peripheral and central vestibular structures. Many ear diseases are associated with vertigo and hearing loss. One of them is Meniere's disease. Careful examination is necessary to differentiate these illnesses from other vestibular disturbances accompanied by vertigo. This study highlighted that neuro-otological examinations in children, especially in small children, is usually more difficult than in adults. The reasons are the extra time involved and the problems connected with a plethora of troublesome individual tests. They agreed that migraine is a common condition in children and can account for some cases of vertigo. Motion sickness is also a common problem that seems to affect the families. One may suspect vertigo in such situations as indeed in many other sensory and perceptive or physical conditions such as visual-spatial problems, deafness or hearing impairment, ineffective and abnormal movements of limbs, tendency to fall, ataxia, behavioural changes and sometimes even clumsiness.

Dyslexia must remain a possible diagnosis in some of these situations particularly if the child has a tendency to bump into objects, difficulty in carrying out daily chores like tying the shoe laces, or locating his room in the house, or failure to do simple spellings, or substituting wrong letters in their writing, etc. Clumsiness is often dubbed as dyslexia, or, worse, retardation, which obviously is a misjudgement. Dyslexia is an established entity that requires specialists in the field to diagnose and manage, on long-term basis. A child suspected of dyslexia must be referred to the relevant specialist.

Head injury is of course an important incident even without the symptoms of nausea or vomiting. It may account for the symptoms of dizziness after a fall. The ear infections particularly chronic ear disease may be an important cause of vertigo in children. Congenital cholesteatoma is rare but must be investigated in a hearing-impaired child with a history of chronic otorrhoea, an attic perforation, an attic retraction pocket, granulation tissue in the pars flaccida or an unusual aural polyp. Children have sometimes presented with facial nerve palsy, mastoiditis, headache, nausea, sickness and dizziness. An intracranial complication is not an unlikely event in some situations.

Metabolic disorders like diabetes particularly the type 1 must be considered an important differential diagnosis in a fainting child. Some immune deficiency disorders and even cytomegalovirus has been incriminated as a possible cause.

BPPV remains relatively underdiagnosed in children. Most clinicians associate BPPV with ageing, though head trauma can also cause it, and should be suspected in children following a head injury. Studied 124 children suffering from vertigo (Mierzwinski et al. 2007). Out of them, 14 had BPPV. Following a clinical examination and vestibular investigations, eight patients were discovered to have abnormal ENG, and the calorimetry showed only one patient to have a canal paresis indicative of a peripheral lesion. Out of these, seven patients had central/mixed pathology. The treatment was symptomatic yielding a satisfactory outcome. It was also noted that a couple of patients after remission developed migraine. The study describes that a follow-up was carried out, in which it was noted that the children suffered from episodic vertigo of variable intensity and frequency. The authors point out that in their view, the childhood BPPV occurred mainly in preschool ages, i.e. 1–7 years. The authors recommended that the older children with the onset of symptoms like BPPV should be suspected for functional background of the disease.

It is a known observation that BPPV does not display any specific findings on an ENG. It was noted by these authors also who reiterate that the only objective evidence of vestibular dysfunction was the presence of nystagmus during the attack. It was also opined that the vascular spasm may have a role to play in many such cases.

We have observed in many children that if interrogated thoroughly, a positive history of headaches intense enough to make them sick or unwell to skip the school for the day may be found. It could well be a mild or moderate migraine, which many toddlers may not be able to express satisfactorily. Even some older children may complain of simple headaches; trying to shun the bright light or a psychedelic light such as the moving colourful pictures on the TV and complaining of sickness should be noted down. As it may well be a form of migraine.

Then, there are many children who simply feel sick on sitting in a moving vehicle. It could well be a simple affair of motion sickness brought about by a rather over sensitive vestibular apparatus. Whether these children need any further in-depth investigations is debateable. We feel that a probing history and a negative clinical examination particularly for a neurological cause may suffice. Some clinicians may, however, prefer to have a negative evidence, if at all, rather than rely upon on their clinical perception and judgment only, as was shown by the following study.

Worden and colleagues (2007) concurred with the popular opinion that evaluation of children with vestibular complaints may be challenging. They agree that the approach to these patients is often quite different than the approach to adults with similar complaints. They believe that the contemporary evidence has elucidated the commonest aetiologies of vertigo in children. Besides, it has documented the utility and feasibility of objective diagnostic tests, e.g. ENG and vestibular-evoked myogenic potentials. More important is the fact that the emerging evidence supports the usefulness of new therapies such as rizatriptan in migraine in children. They summarised that an evidence-based approach to the evaluation of paediatric vestibular dysfunction may improve diagnostic yield and facilitate timely initiation of appropriate therapy. And that to say the least would be an achievement that should grant relief to the patient and his family and much gratification to the physician. It goes without saying that in all patients, but particularly in children, the time is of the essence. Prompt and correct diagnosis followed by most suitable treatment is the objective of all physicians across the board. It has been the motto since time immemorial and is the fundamental rule of ethics, i.e. beneficence.

It was noted by Bencsik et al. (2007) that pathologies from childhood to adolescence carry physical, cognitive, motor, linguistic, perceptual, social, emotional and neurosensory characteristics. The ages between 8 and 15 especially carry very special traits of a rollover in data processing with respect to the maintenance of balance and postural control. Data acquisition of neuro-otological function provided them with a network of information about the sensory status of their young patients. In their view, major neuro-otological complaint leading to functional neuro-otological investigations is vertigo with or without nausea, etc. These complaints may present as acute vertigo but may also be chronic and relapsing.

This study is extremely useful as it clearly defines certain observable, tangible clinical features which may in fact be called the cardinal principles of diagnosis of paediatric vertigo. They are described as the physiological and clinical syndromes displaying a combination of four principal phenomena:

(a) Perceptual (vertigo).
(b) Oculomotor (nystagmus).
(c) Postural (dystaxia).
(d) Vegetative (nausea, vomiting).

These four manifestations of vertigo appear to be related to different levels of the vestibular involvement, requiring different methods of investigation. The focus of their study was the phase of restructuring of balance control in children between the ages of 8 and 15 years.

Obviously matters of neuro-otological manifestations deserve much closer and deeper analysis by a neurologist. It is therefore a common clinical practice that such children (and adults) are immediately referred to the neurologists for a comprehensive checkup.

The following article duly manifests the importance of urgent evaluation and prompt referral of neuro-otological emergencies.

Seemungal (2007) agreed with the general observation that most physicians find acute vertigo a diagnostic challenge, particularly in children. This article reviewed recent evidence outlining the clinical presentation of acute central and peripheral dizzy syndromes and suggests the time, when a clinician may consider imaging. All clinicians know of the difficulty that acute vertigo may pose, sometimes. The author quotes several practical illustrations of our dilemmas. For instance, migrainous vertigo may have oculomotor abnormalities suggestive of either central neurological or peripheral vestibular dysfunction. A case of vertebrobasilar artery insufficiency in an adult may mimic a peripheral disorder such as vestibular neuronitis. Or indeed if it is associated with hearing loss, it may be misdiagnosed as Meniere's disease. The author believed that the recent evidences have not made the assessment of acute vertigo any easier for the nonspecialist. Although the common causes of vertigo are simple and easily manageable, serious conditions such as a stroke may be mistaken for a peripheral vestibulopathy. Conversely, benign conditions such as migrainous vertigo may have clinical characteristics of central disorders. These findings re-emphasise the need for a thorough clinical evaluation of the acutely dizzy patient. There is so much overlap in the symptomatology that the diagnosis of vertigo may prove to be a conundrum, especially for someone not dealing with it on a daily basis.

The point made in this paper needs no further emphasis except that the diagnosis of vertigo in children is significantly more challenging than in adults. Furthermore, in a toddler, it is often complex, sometimes with multiple symptoms; hence, referral to a neurologist should not be delayed.

Abuse of antibiotics is a common practice in many parts of the world. The oto-toxic drugs particularly the aminoglycoside group must be considered as a possible cause in a patient who may have travelled from one of the developing countries. TB is still a force to reckon with in Africa and parts of Asia, and streptomycin is the drug of choice in many such nations. Children given either streptomycin or one of its variants may suffer not only with vertigo but also with severe to profound degree of hearing loss along with most disturbing tinnitus.

Aminoglycoside eardrops are commonly used in many counties in discharging ears with perforated eardrums. It is debateable if the amount of the aminoglycoside absorbed by the middle ear mucosa in such situations can be large enough to cause any serious internal area problem; however, cumulative effects of drugs is not unknown to cause many untoward side effects.

Many neurological conditions like cerebral palsy, hydrocephalus, Wallenberg's lateral medullary syndrome and even malignant tumours of the brain are not unknown in children and are obviously important causes of dizziness. Cerebellar ataxia is an important factor that must always be kept in mind in a child who staggers to take a few steps in the right direction. We find it an extremely useful observation to watch carefully as the child enters the consulting room and behaves in and around the objects in the clinic, while we are taking the history from mum. If he tends to veer to a side or bumph into objects, a quiet note is made in the mind until a clinical examination is carried out. Simple tests like the Romberg's and the Unterberger's test are easy to perform on children and can give considerable information about the vestibulo-oculo-cerebellar integrity or otherwise.

Childhood depression is said to be an important factor too, particularly in the current culture of bullying and harassment at schools. Maternal intoxication with drugs, alcoholism (foetal alcoholic syndrome), broken homes, battered babies and trauma inflicted upon the babies are reported on the British National Television on almost daily basis. Obviously the least such psychologically traumatising experience can do to the child is give a him a constant and nagging headache with dizziness, sickness, despair, depression and hopelessness.

During the seasonal variations particularly in bad winter months, viral infections are known to dominate our lives, as was seen with the swine flu a few years ago. Therefore, it is not unusual to find a bout of viral labyrinthitis or vestibular neuronitis in children. Although this discussion is mainly confined to vestibular causes, one should still not forget numerous congenital cardio-vascular conditions that may account for a vast number of children presenting with symptoms of vertigo, presyncope, syncope, etc. History remains the touch stone in the process of diagnosis of vertigo.

Children have their own ways of presenting their complaints. A famous paediatrician once said that children are not young adults. Infants, babies and toddlers have their own anatomical, physiological, biochemical, psychological and pathological profiles. Weiss and Phillips (2006) mention similarities in clinical conditions but also duly highlighted the differences between children and the adults in this study. They observed that paediatric neurologists see many children with vestibular disorders. Some of them present with acute vestibular symptoms; others may have migraine-related vertigo, benign positional vertigo, basilar migraine, cyclic vomiting, etc. Meniere's may be seen in some children, even a perilymph fistula. They also reported five children with previously unrecognised vestibular dysfunction detected clinically and confirmed through vestibular testing. One child had fluctuating visual acuity with intermittent nystagmus. Another child had episodic vertigo with congenital hearing loss and imbalance; the third had neurotrophic keratitis, imbalance and motor delays. Another child presented with ataxia and abnormal eye movement following head injury. The fifth child had episodic vertigo and eye movements' abnormalities from infancy. In this study, a quantitative vestibular testing was carried out through dynamic visual acuity, post-head shake nystagmus and computerised platform posturography. They mention that paediatric neurologists do encounter children with congenital nystagmus and compensated vestibular dysfunction in their clinics, which can be recognised on the basis of history and clinical examination such as abnormalities of the vestibulo-ocular reflex. Obviously in these patients, a firm diagnosis would require a detailed investigation. Unlike adults, many children may not be able to express their symptoms accurately enough. It is therefore essential that as an otolaryngologist, close link-up may be maintained with the paediatrician regarding any significant contributors to the menace of vertigo. We have a huge advantage in our clinics where we are ably supported and guided by an excellent community paediatrician, which is a blessing in many ways.

Not only does it help us in getting a real picture of the problem, but as team, we can serve our children much better than would do otherwise.

In the early 1960s, stapedectomy proved to be magical and quite a melodramatic procedure. Stapedectomy in children, however, was a highly controversial and an unpopular practice. The surgeons knew that the process of otosclerosis is metabolic, and the artificial prosthesis would not stop it from involving the cochlea at some stage, a condition aptly called the cochlear otosclerosis. It applied to adults also. But in children, it was particularly relevant to avoid stapedectomy, because the life of the prosthesis was usually no more than a few years. It obviously meant the replacement of the prosthesis at a later stage in his life. Surgeons also knew that even in the best of hands 2 % of the patients following stapedectomy could end up with dead cochlea. So the practice never caught on. Of course now the hearing aid technology is so advanced that surgery has practically no role to play in these cases.

If they had found a perfect ossicular prosthesis, the innovative gadgets that are still being promoted would have not seen the light of the day. So the search goes on.

Deafness is another matter. The cochlear implants have indeed revolutionised the management of a deaf person. In children, it has definitely made much difference to the overall burden of disability and disease in the last couple of decades. Not all cochlear implants go smoothly, though, as complications ensuing an implant are not an unknown entity. One such problem could be witnessed in the form of imbalance. In some cases, vestibular impairment has followed a cochlear implant.

Having said that one must hasten to add that until the day that stem cell research reaches a stage, when a nerve cell and a cochlea may be cultivated or regenerated through eugenics, it appears that the cochlear implant is no less than a biblical panacea for a deaf child. But even such panaceas are known to have side effects!

Cochlear implant is a miracle of the recent times. It has changed the life of innumerable deaf persons and continues to do with ever-gaining popularity. One must, however, remember that the cochlear loss may also be associated with a vestibular impairment.

Cochlear implants are becoming increasingly popular, and many more centres are carrying out these procedures than in the past decade. Some of these potential candidates for implants may have either unilateral or bilateral vestibular involvement also. This subject is not duly highlighted as it should be. Jacot et al. (2009) looked at the prevalence and types of vestibular impairments in sensorineural hearing loss, in a large population of paediatric candidates for cochlear implants. This research involved 224 children with profound SNHL who underwent complete vestibular testing before the implantation of a cochlear implant. Following the implants, changes in vestibular responses were measured in 89 of them. It was noted that in the SNHL population, only 50 % had normal bilateral vestibular function, while 20 % had bilateral complete areflexia, 22.5 % had partial asymmetrical hypoexcitability and 7.5 % had partial symmetrical hypoexcitability. In a vast majority of follow-up patients showing vestibular responses prior to implant, 51 (71 %) had changes in vestibular function including 7 (10 %) who demonstrated ipsilateral areflexia. Other patients developed ipsilateral hypo- or hyperexcitability. It was also observed that vestibular modifications occurred during the 3 months after surgery and were not clearly associated with clinical signs except for ipsilateral areflexia. The good news was that after a long-term follow-up, two of the seven patients with ipsilateral areflexia partially recovered their vestibular function.

They concluded that since half of paediatric cochlear implant candidates had vestibular deficits and 51 % of implants induced modifications of existing vestibular function, each implant should be preceded by canal and otolith functional tests to ensure that the ear with the least functional vestibule is implanted.

This study is of great value to a cochlear implants team, as it provides a useful guideline. A vestibulometry prior to implants should provide baselines for follow-up and active monitoring.

The diagnosis of vertigo in children, particular those with profound SNHL, is challenging and demands considerable patience on the part of the physician.

A similar study is mentioned here for comparison in adult patients. Melvin et al. (2009) investigated the risk posed by cochlear implantation to the labyrinth. Thirty-six ears in 35 adult cochlear implant candidates were investigated. They looked at the vestibular function, using the quantitative 3-dimensional head impulse test (qHIT), clinical head impulse test (cHIT), post-head shake nystagmus, caloric elect-ronystagmography, vestibular-evoked myogenic potentials, dynamic visual acuity and Dizziness Handicap Inventory. By any standards, one might say, they were rather detailed and highly reliable studies with proven specificity and sensitivity.

The conclusion of the study was that although small, the observed rate of laby-rinthine injury was comparable to that for other risks of a cochlear implant. It is important, the authors believe, to warn in some detail the candidates for cochlear implants regarding the possible risk to vestibular function, particularly when the implantation of an 'only functioning vestibular side' is contemplated. They also found the head impulse test a useful clinical tool particularly for picking up severe high-frequency vestibular hypofunction, and they believe it should form part of the pre-cochlear implant physical examination. One cannot not argue with that. We feel that this simple clinical test is an invaluable tool and is currently underemployed.

The development of the vestibular and the cochlear components of the ear is intimate and can go wrong, resulting in the congenital or developmental errors of either or both parts. Cushing et al. (2008) believe that embryological and anatomical similarities between the auditory and vestibular systems suggest that children with sensorineural hearing loss (SNHL) may demonstrate vestibular impairments. This hypothesis was therefore tested in 40 children with severe to profound SNHL and a history of unilateral cochlear implants. In these children, vestibular function was assessed with caloric, rotational and vestibular-evoked myogenic potential testing. Furthermore, their balance was assessed using the balance subset of the Bruininks–Oseretsky Test of Motor Proficiency-II, which is a standardised test of static and dynamic balance.

These workers found out that the function of the horizontal semicircular canal was abnormal in response to a caloric stimulus in 50 % (16/32), with a large propor-tion of those (6/16 (38 %)) reflecting mild to moderate unilateral abnormalities. In comparison, horizontal semicircular canal function in response to rotation was abnormal in 38 % (14/37). Saccular function was absent bilaterally in 5/26 (19 %) and unilaterally in 5/26 (19 %) with vestibular-evoked myogenic potential. SNHL from meningitis was associated with worse balance function than other aetiologies.

It was therefore inferred that vestibular and balance dysfunction occurred in >1/3 of children with SNHL and cochlear implants and is highly dependent on aetiology. Although compliance with all tests was high, rotational chair testing, which assesses higher frequency motion (0.25–5 Hz) and thus more 'real-world' vestibular function, correlated best with dynamic balance. For this reason, they believe that rotational chair testing may represent the test of choice in this population, particularly given that it is amenable to testing children of all ages.

Congenital deafness is a major issue globally but more so in the developing countries, particularly in some African and many Asian countries. In the Muslim population, consanguineous marriages are not only a norm but actually encouraged due to tribal, traditional and cultural reasons (Zaidi 2000). In the Muslim population in Britain, congenital, hereditary, syndromal and asyndromal deafness continues to pose a challenge.

Vestibular function may or may not be affected in children born with a syndromal or asyndromal type of deafness. It is a subject that is somewhat underinvestigated. Kaga et al. (2008), however, showed that congenitally deaf children commonly suffer from vestibular failure in both ears. They also noted that the development of gross motor functions such as head control, sitting and walking is likely to be delayed, but fine motor function is usually preserved unless disorders of the central nervous system are concomitantly present. More importantly, such children can eventually catch up with their normal peers in terms of development and growth due to the central vestibular compensation. The visual and somatosensory systems, pyramidal and extrapyramidal motor system (cerebellum, basal ganglia) and intellectual development are known to compensate for vestibular failure in these babies. Therefore, thanks to the compensatory mechanisms, these children grow up fairly normally.

Expensive and time-consuming imaging techniques may not be required as often as many clinicians do. In a contemporary study by Wiener-Vacher (2008), it was duly reiterated that vertigo in a child is a matter of great concern for the physician and the family. They concur that often enough prior to a comprehensive otological, neurological and vestibular/clinical examination, physicians may request a CT or MRI scanning, when in most cases such expensive investigations could be unnecessary.

This work was based on the results of a 14-year study conducted with a sample of more than 2,000 children referred for balance disorders to the functional vestibular evaluation unit of the ENT paediatric department in Paris. The clinical signs of vestibular deficit and the most frequent aetiologies of vertigo and dizziness in children were identified as migraine equivalent, ophthalmologic disorders, benign paroxysmal idiopathic paediatric vertigo and temporal bone fracture.

Posterior fossa tumours are fortunately rare to occur, forming less than 1 % of total cases of juvenile vertigo. These tumours present with ataxia and are usually seen by neurologists. Clinically though, from an ENT point of view, it is essential to keep this condition in mind, as an important differential diagnosis if the child presents with cerebellar signs, torticollis, cranial nerve involvement such as of the oculomotor nerve, hemianopia, unilateral hypotonia or Babinski's sign. An MRI scan and urgent involvement of a neuro-otologist or a neurosurgeon is needed. Children are very susceptible to serious problems; therefore, one must be extra cautious and arrange for an urgent review by the neurologist or a neurotologist in a suspected case.

Acoustic neuroma is an extremely rare tumour in the paediatric age group, as it is a naturally slow-growing tumour and may take years to present itself as cause of vertigo.

No doubt every paediatric otolaryngologist feels highly concerned indeed engaged in establishing the cause of vestibular pathology, if any, in a child who presents with dizziness. It is not always easy to reach a final diagnosis, despite the comprehensive investigations. The clinician must not leave any stone unturned in carrying out thorough clinical and vestibular, imaging and other pertinent investigations to reach a definitive decision. It was duly highlighted by Nandi and Luxon (2008) in a study. They reminded us that the vestibular system develops from 'optic placode', an embryonic ectodermal thickening located on either side of the developing neural tube near the formative hindbrain in the primitive pharynx. The future vestibular organ develops, from a specialised structure called the 'otocysts'. From this structure, the membranous and the vestibular labyrinth develop.

These authors have described a systematic approach to the management of a vertiginous child. It is an exceedingly useful paper that all clinicians dealing with vertigo must read and apply the knowledge thus gained in their practical life. Once again, history taking is on top of their list also, followed by a comprehensive clinical examination. In a child, these authors recommend a comprehensive maternal history taking. It is extremely important such as the nature of pregnancy, gestation period, any exposure to viral infections, drug toxicity, duration of labour and any incidents involved such as an undue delay, trauma and hypoxia. It should be followed by a history of developmental mile stones, delay in crawling, sitting, standing, tendency to fall, inability to turn from his side, etc. All must be documented. Developmental history should extend beyond the early stages to the present day.

Luxon and Nandi advocate the use of simple observations such as the facial deformities or malformed external ears as a low-set early cup-shaped pinnae may indicate Down's or Goldenhar syndrome. They also recommend the use of a video camera attached to a purpose built camera. One must also exclude characters seen in CHARGE with choanal atresia as it may be associated with semicircular agenesis. They also discuss many clinical and audio-vestibular tests such as an observation of nystagmus, Hamalgyi head thrust, head shake nystagmus, dynamic visual acuity, Dix–Hallpike test, gait assessment and neuro-otological examination. Vestibular investigations are also discussed by these authors at length, such as calorimetry, rotational testing, posturography and VEMPs. Some of these tests are described in this clinical guide.

They pointed out that paediatric vestibular assessment is necessary in various situations, yielding invaluable information for the diagnosis, and for appropriate rehabilitative strategies in the management of children with vestibular and balance problems, alone or in association with hearing impairment or other developmental disorders. No one can argue the point made by these authors. It duly highlights the significance of the detailed and thorough investigation in children presenting with vertigo.

Paediatric vertigo is an undermanaged clinical problem. Once established, many children will benefit with standard medical or sometimes surgical interventions as discussed elsewhere in this monograph. Some, however, may require rehabilitations therapy.

This mode of treatment was studied by Medeiros et al. (2005). Through clinical assessment and computerised dynamic posturography, they investigated the outcome of children with peripheral vestibular disturbances undergoing vestibular rehabilitation therapy and observed the influence of learning and of central nervous system maturation on posturography retest results. Sixteen symptomatic children underwent pre-and posttreatment computerised dynamic posturography compared with matching cohorts as controls. They describe various vestibular rehab exercises consisting of a series of physical exercises that include eye, head and various body movements, with the objective of stimulating the vestibular, somatosensory and visual systems. They have identified relevant exercises, described as sitting with head still and eye movements in different positions or head movements, from side to side or forward backwards movements, etc. Specific details of such exercises are available in relevant manuals.

The outcome was clinically assessed. The workers noted that all children completed the treatment. Total recovery of symptoms occurred in approximately 53 % of the patients, whereas a dramatic partial recovery was observed in majority of other children. No adverse reactions occurred to the exercises. Furthermore, no statistically significant posturography changes were observed in the asymptomatic children. It was therefore concluded that the vestibular rehabilitation therapy seems to be a safe and efficacious therapeutic option in children with peripheral vestibular disturbances.

Worden and Blevins (2007) observed that evaluation of children with vestibular complaints may be challenging. It was opined that the approach to these patients is often quite different compared to the adults with similar complaints. The authors suggested that the recent evidence has elucidated the commonest aetiologies of vertigo in children, documented the utility and feasibility of objective diagnostic testing such as electronystagmography and vestibular-evoked myogenic potentials in this population and demonstrated the efficacy of new therapies such as rizatriptan for the treatment of migraine in children. It was therefore summarised that an evidence-based approach to the evaluation of paediatric vestibular dysfunction may improve diagnostic yield and facilitate timely initiation of appropriate therapy.

No one can disagree with this proposal by the authors as the current practice of medicine is certainly evidence based. They also pointed out that the pathologies from childhood to adolescence carry physical, cognitive, motor, linguistic, perceptual, social, emotional and neurosensory characteristics. That is certainly an observation that most clinicians would agree with. The trauma whether physical or psychological borne by a person in the formative years leaves permanent marks on human psyche.

The treatment of vertigo in children varies between symptomatic anti-vertiginous drugs given only if needed to vestibular rehabilitation therapy. Currently the emphasis is mainly upon rehab exercise carried out under the expert supervision of the vestibular therapists or under their advice to be pursued at home. Its usefulness is constantly being monitored by the clinicians.

Teggi et al. (2009) assessed the efficacy of rehabilitation for dizzy patients after the recent acute vestibular disturbance in 40 patients. They randomly divided them into two groups. Half of them underwent active rehabilitation, while the other half were instructed to perform the routine daily activities only. After 25 days, the rehabilitated patients were seen to record better results for all recorded outcomes. It was a very sensitive and scientifically sound study in which Teggi et al. (2009) showed the effectiveness of a supervised exercise programme for patients with acute vestibular disturbance. No doubt, in their view, a good rehabilitation programme reduces dependence on visual cues for maintenance of posture and its effective control.

It is a common experience that children with vertigo may have other associated clinical conditions also. That should be addressed simultaneously, such as errors of refraction or a strabismus, physical deformities and sometimes neurological deficits requiring referral to the dedicated neurological clinics.

Vestibular therapy is proving to have an important role to play in the management of postural vertigo. Visual-motor control, rehab exercises and many other practices adopted in our setup as indeed elsewhere are discussed in the chapter on vestibular rehabilitation. The study proved the point that vestibular rehab therapy is quite helpful in managing the children with peripheral vestibular lesions.

There is no doubt that majority of vertiginous children respond to medical treatment better than adults. Some may, however, need short- or long-term vestibular rehab therapy.

Many clinicians agree that vestibulopathies form a major cause of vertigo in children. Such children may present with a wide variety of symptoms as discussed before. Clinically one can diagnose most, but some require further investigations to arrive at a definite diagnosis. Most vestibulopathies resolve naturally, tough rehab exercises expedite the recovery. Bittar et al. (2002) prospectively analysed 22 children with vestibulopathy treated with vestibular rehabilitation employing Cawthorne and Cooksey's methods. They employed ENG and rotational chair as the tests for vestibular functions, though a history of vestibular disorder was accepted despite the normal tests. Their results showed that all the patients improved. They claim that vestibular rehabilitation is a therapeutic alternative in children. We feel that unwanted medication should be avoided, instead vestibular rehabilitation may be advised.

In conclusion, one is obliged to agree with most workers who have advocated extreme attention to detailed history, clinical examination and vestibular investigations as well as imaging, in vertiginous children. No one can doubt nor underplay the psychological and emotional factors that nearly always dominate the presentation and management of a vertigo inflicted child. Parental anxiety in such situations is often overbearing and may have an adverse effect on the decision-making. It is important that the management of a dizzy child should involve a multidisciplinary approach. The family physician obviously has the basic role to play, but involvement of a paediatrician and neurologists at an appropriate time must also be kept in mind. Long-term management of such a child usually is medicinal and rehabilitative with positive outcomes. Dilated vestibular aqueduct syndrome is a rare condition mostly detected in early life.

It is extremely rare to find a case of a dilated vestibular aqueduct in an adult. They are usually diagnosed in early childhood. Manzari (2008) defines the function of the aqueduct and the sac as the agents responsible for endolymphatic homeostasis, immune defence of the inner ear and elimination of endolymphatic debris. This is indeed a novel explanation, but close to logic. Therefore, it is understandable that its abnormality either development or acquired will lead to vertigo or vertiginous symptoms. It was also mentioned by Manzari that a dilated vestibular aqueduct system may present as instability or recurring oscillopsia, lowered vestibular EMG potential, hypoacusis, a history of migraine-related vertigo or motion sickness and a nystagmus induced by mastoid vibration and head shake test and VOR gain elevation on rotational chair testing. In this study, they investigated a number of cases to identify a pattern of signs and symptoms as well as neurological findings which would assist an investigation of vestibular function in patients with anatomical variation of the duct and sac. In this unusual study, 15 subjects affected by volumetric abnormalities of the vestibular aqueduct were selected from a cohort of patients referred to a tertiary referral neuro-otological centre. All the patients underwent accurate clinical history taking and were evaluated using a standardised set of bedside and instrumental neuro-otological tests, namely, the audiometry, ABR and vestibular-evoked myogenic potentials. Following which, each patient had a CT and an MR imaging in order to accurately evaluate the middle and the inner ear.

These evaluations confirmed a clinical suspicion of volumetric abnormalities of the vestibular aqueduct and endolymphatic sac.

It also demonstrated that all patients with a defined volumetric alteration in the region of the vestibular aqueduct and endolymphatic sac had very typical clinical presentation. The most obvious and frequent symptoms in these patients were vestibular migraine (using the Neuhauser criteria) affecting 66.6 %, 'motion sickness' in 80 %, oscillopsia in 60 % and dizziness per se in 93.3 %.

The clinical examinations for the selected patients allowed some useful speculative conclusions. They found that the vestibular-evoked myogenic potentials of the neck, and the mastoid vibration test at 100 Hz, were extremely useful diagnostic aids.

Manzari, therefore, concluded that dysfunction of the vestibular aqueduct is suggested by symptomatology characterised by a history of vestibular migraine, unstable or recurring oscillopsia, a fall in the vestibular-evoked myogenic potential threshold, hypoacusis and nystagmus induced by mastoid vibration and head shaking. The author believed that imaging is of immense value to confirm the clinical suspicions. These clinical indicators and diagnostic factors are worthy of note.

Such studies are highly innovative and extremely helpful both for the clinician as well as research scientists. This study certainly deserves merit and demands that many other similar investigations may be carried out, basically to outline the relevant parameters and identify the variables in patients presenting with unusual symptoms. Anatomical and morphological changes in the inner ear can thus be identified through the investigations mentioned by Manzari. Textbooks of anatomy are inundated with various embryological and morphological variants in the ear. Some of them have specific names like the Mondini, Pendred, Treacher Collins and Moon–Biedl syndromes. We have seen most of them in our hearing services. Anyone interested in more detailed description of such syndromes may refer to a standard ENT textbook.

References

Abu-Arafeh I, Russell G (1995) Paroxysmal vertigo as migraine equivalent in children: a population based study. Cephalalgia 15(1):22–25

Aust G, Novotny M (2005) Meniere's disease and various types of vertigo in children. Int Tinnitus J 11(1):66–68, 0946–5448

Bencsik B, Bencze G, Nagy E, Heid L, Claussen CF (2007) Neuro-otological aspects of juvenile vertigo. Int Tinnitus J 13(1):57–62, 0946–5448

Berrettini S, Forli F, Bogazzi F, Neri E, Salvatori L, Casani AP, Franceschini SS (2005) Large vestibular aqueduct syndrome: audiological, radiological, clinical, and genetic features. Am J Otolaryngol 26(6):363–371, 0196–0709

Bittar RSM, Pedalini MEB, Medeiros IRT, Bottino MA, Bento RF (2002) Vestibular rehabilitation in children: preliminary study. Rev Bras Otorrinolaringol 68(4):496–499, 0034–7299

Cushing SL, Papsin BC, Rutka JA, James AL, Gordon KA (2008) Evidence of vestibular and balance dysfunction in children with profound sensorineural hearing loss using cochlear implants. Laryngoscope 118(10):1814–1823, 0023–852X; 1531–4995

Eviatar L, Eviatar A (1977) Vertigo in children: differential diagnosis and treatment. Pediatrics 59:833–838

Fried MP (1980) The evaluation of dizziness in children. Laryngoscopes 90:1548–1560

Jacot E, Van Den Abbeele T, Debre HR, Wiener-Vacher SR (2009) Vestibular impairments pre- and post-cochlear implant in children. Int J Pediatr Otorhinolaryngol 73(2):209–217, 0165–5876

Kaga K, Shinjo Y, Jin Y, Takegoshi H (2008) Vestibular failure in children with congenital deafness. Int J Audiol 47(9):590–599, 1499–2027; 1708–8186

Maki-Torkko E, Magnusson M (2005) An office procedure to detect vestibular loss in children with hearing impairment. Eur Arch Otorhinolaryngol 262(4):328–330, 0937–4477

Manzari L (2008) Vestibular signs and symptoms of volumetric abnormalities of the vestibular aqueduct. J Laryngol Otol 122(6):557–563

Medeiros IRT, Bittar RSM, Pedalini MEB, Lorenzi MC, Formigoni LG, Bento RF (2005) Vestibular rehabilitation therapy in children. Otol Neurotol 26(4):699–703, 1531–7129; 1537–4505

Melvin TA, Della Santina CC, Carey JP, Migliaccio AA (2009) The effects of cochlear implantation on vestibular function. Otol Neurotol 30(1):87–94, 1531–7129; 1537–4505

Mierzwinski J, Polak M, Dalke K, Burduk P, Kazmierczak H, Modrzynski M (2007) Benign paroxysmal vertigo of childhood. Otolaryngol Pol 61(3):307–310, 0030–6657

Nandi R, Luxon LM (2008) Development and assessment of the vestibular system. Int J Audiol 47(9):566–577

Niemensivu R, Pyykko I, Wiener-Vacher SR, Kentala E (2006) Vertigo and balance problems in children – an epidemiologic study in Finland. Int J Paediatr Otorhinolaryngol 70(2): 259–265

Seemungal BM (2007) Neuro-otological emergencies. Curr Opin Neurol 20(1):32–39, 1350–7540; 1080–8248

Teggi R, Caldiroal D, Fabiano B, Recanti P, Bussi M (2009) Rehabilitation after acute vestibular disorders. J Laryngol Otol 123(4):397–402, 0022–2151; 1748–5460

Weiss AH, Phillips JO (2006) Congenital and compensated vestibular dysfunction in childhood: an overlooked entity. J Child Neurol 21(7):572–579

Wiener-Vacher SR (2008) Vestibular disorders in children. Int J Audiol 47(9):578–583, 1499–2027; 1708–8186

Worden BF, Blevins NH (2007) Paediatric vestibulopathy and pseudovestibulopathy: differential diagnosis and management. Curr Opin Otolaryngol Head Neck Surg 15(5):304–309, 1068–9508

Zaidi SH (2000) Deafness in the developing nations. Royal Book Co., Karachi

Part III

Rehabilitation and Ethical Issues

Rehabilitation

11

Many cases of vertigo respond satisfactorily to therapeutic management either medically or surgically. Some may, however, remain refractory to any form of treatment. Others may only need rehabilitative measures.

A common example of therapeutic management of vertigo is a case of cholesteatoma. Once treated surgically, the patient is duly rewarded with not only safety of life, which is the prime object of tympano-mastoid surgery, but also remains free of vertiginous symptoms. Dizziness in these cases is usually a sign of CSOM encroaching upon the delicate labyrinthine capsule sometimes resulting in labyrinthitis. After eradication of the disease with tympano-mastoid surgery, these patients find much relief in carrying out their daily chores.

An example where therapeutic management is neither indicated nor fruitful is that of BPPV. Before the advent of Epley's manoeuvre, these patients really suffered with long-term instability in posture, positional dizziness and worst of all fear of fall and insecurity. Epley's manoeuvre has changed all that and made life simple and restored the quality of life to these patients, which was otherwise compromised.

Epley's manoeuvre is a fine example of rehabilitative measure that a clinician can perform. It is simple, least time-consuming, economical and highly gratifying to both, i.e. the patient and the clinician.

One major problem seen in day-to-day practice is that of long-term use of anti-vertiginous drugs. It is to be condemned with the strongest words, as the vestibular compensatory mechanism is duly insulted and considerably slowed down with such a practice. Such drugs should be used only on short-term basis, basically to provide instant relief from acute vertigo. The prophylactic use of many drugs may have no more than a placebo effect, in most situations.

Following an acute attack of vertigo, the central nervous system immediately comes into action. Due measures are initiated to enable the labyrinth overcome the trauma or damage, just like it happens physiologically in other bodily injuries. The compensatory mechanism commences and continues until the labyrinth recovers. It happens slowly and gradually, but if medication is given for a prolonged period of time, the central compensatory mechanism becomes lazy and allows the labyrinth to respond to the drugs. That means the natural recovery time is unduly prolonged.

S.H. Zaidi, A. Sinha, *Vertigo*,
DOI 10.1007/978-3-642-36485-3_11, © Springer-Verlag Berlin Heidelberg 2013

This does not mean that an acute case of vertigo may be allowed to suffer while the central systems take over the control, far from it. What it means is that clinically judging the patients' symptoms once the acute stage has settled down with drugs, the clinician should gradually reduce and finally withdraw the medication.

The efficacy of vestibular rehabilitation with the electrotactile-vestibular substitution system, as a new treatment modality in patients with bilateral vestibular disorders (Polat et al. 2010), was investigated. Nineteen patients with bilateral, chronic, idiopathic vestibulopathy were divided in two groups. The first group was rehabilitated with the electrotactile-vestibular substitution system, while the second group was treated with standard vestibular rehabilitation therapy. The sensory organisation test and dizziness handicap inventory were used to compare the pre- and post-training results of both rehabilitative treatments. It was observed that all patients in the first group demonstrated improved results for both the composite sensory organisation test and for the functional transfer aspect of the dizziness handicap inventory, after 5 days' training with the electrotactile-vestibular substitution system. In contrast, group two patients showed no significant improvement in their composite sensory organisation test or dizziness handicap inventory scores after 8 weeks of therapy, compared with pre-treatment levels. These workers believe that these preliminary results indicate the efficacy of the electrotactile-vestibular substitution system in improving patients' symptoms of vestibulopathy and constitute evidence of successful sensory substitution. Further research is obviously needed in this regard.

Childs (2010) noted that the patients with unilateral vestibular hypofunction can be treated using adaptation, substitution and exercises. Patients with motion sensitivity can demonstrate improved tolerance to motion after performing habituation exercises. Patients with bilateral vestibular loss will benefit from substitution and adaptation exercises. Each patient requires a treatment regime that is customised to meet the individual needs. Often the treatment is determined through the evaluation process. The task that causes the patient's complaints, whether it is dizziness, imbalance and/or issues with eye–head coordination, often becomes the treatment of choice, gradually increasing difficulty as appropriate and safe.

Patients with transient brain ischaemia (TBI) who have concomitant vestibular dysfunction are a challenging population to treat. One has to be aware of cognitive deficits that may interfere with or prolong the treatment. Most such cases are dealt by the physicians or neurologists; however, some have presented to us in our routine clinics with the symptoms of light-headedness, dizziness and even vertigo. Besides, many other neurological deficits may be present because of the brain injury. For example, attempting to perform the canalith repositioning manoeuvre on a post-TBI patient when he may not be able to comprehend the reasoning behind the treatment can lead to agitation or behavioural issues. Communication with the patient's primary doctor is essential, so that the team is always on the same page about the approach to treatment.

Vestibular evaluation and rehabilitation are a necessity for patients who have experienced a TBI. The sooner the problems are identified, the sooner the treatment can be initiated with the goal of helping patients recover their maximal functional level of independence and safety. One may remember that treating the patients with

TBI and vestibular impairments may require more treatment time when compared to a patient with vestibular disorder alone.

Virk and McConville (2006) reiterate that maintaining balance under all conditions is an absolute requirement for humans. Any degree of imbalance can deeply affect an individual's daily life. They also agreed that orientation in space and maintenance of balance require inputs from the vestibular, the visual, the proprioceptive and the somatosensory systems. All cues coming from these systems are integrated by the central nervous system (CNS) to employ different strategies for orientation and balance. How the CNS integrates all the inputs and makes cognitive decisions about balance strategies has been an area of interest for biomedical engineers for a long time. More interesting is the fact that in the absence of one or more cues, or when the input from one of the sensors is skewed, the CNS 'adapts' to the new environment and gives less weight to the conflicting inputs. It is simply mind boggling to say the least!

The role of neocerebellum is known to the clinicians that it filters out the necessary from the unnecessary sensory information and guides the motor cortex to take an action. In other words it 'prioritises' the information for the higher centres to take a prompt action or postpone it.

Somehow, the neocerebellum does not receive its due recognition and its placement in the order of organs that control the balance. Imagine a clinical situation where the information sent by the peripheral receptors is either deficient or insufficient, due to a malfunctioning neocerebellum. The cerebral cortex will not know whether it is the snake on a country path at dusk, in the way of the traveller, or a piece of rope. The former may be harmful and the later can be safely ignored. It is the neocerebellum that determines the necessity of feeding the requisite information to the motor cortex at an appropriate time. In the elderly folks, it is a common observation that they hesitate to take a step forward if the exteroceptive receptors feed an information about the change in the texture of the ground. Neocerebellum provides the necessary information, based upon the correct information received from the optical sources. It is this harmony of numerous apparently independent elements, coming in motion as a rhythmical, organised and coordinated activity, that controls the posture. Some of the sensory or the motor elements in this orchestra may either malfunction or underperform, thus leading to ataxia, disequilibrium and imbalance.

In their paper, they carried out a review of different strategies and models put forward by researchers to explain the integration of the sensory cues mentioned above. Furthermore, they compared the different approaches used by young and old adults in maintaining the balance. Since the musculoskeletal, visual and vestibular systems deteriorate with age, the older subjects have to compensate for these impaired sensory cues for postural stability. Their paper also discussed the applications of virtual reality in rehabilitation programmes not only for balance in the elderly but also in occupational falls. Virtual reality has profound applications in the field of balance rehabilitation and training because of its relatively low cost.

Further studies should be conducted to evaluate the effectiveness of 'virtual reality training' in modifying the head and eye movement strategies and determine the role of these responses in the maintenance of balance.

Case Report

Mrs. P was born in 1920 and presented to our vestibular lab for investigation of her vertigo. She reported a fall a few months ago and believed that she might have lost her consciousness. She was taken to the A/E department by an ambulance. She said that though she still felt dizzy, but has not lost consciousness since the first episode, she had to walk with a stick to support herself. She had a constant fear of fall. She denied any veering to right or left. She said she had to steady herself on the side of her bed before getting up to walk as she had fallen back on to the bed on a few occasions while getting out of it. She denied any rotatory vertigo but noticed a sensation of movement in her head occurring a few times a day. She reported some dizziness on bending forward but not on rolling over in bed or looking up. She said that her confidence is shaken up and she found her quality of life greatly compromised.

Mrs. P felt that she heard better on the left side and was quite comfortable with her hearing aids which were recently readjusted at the hearing services. She thought that her hearing loss was noise induced due to exposure at war. She noticed occasional tinnitus which was not bothersome. She had hypertension controlled with drugs and took thyroxin for hypothyroidism. She was referred for an MRI scan and awaited results.

The otoscopy was normal. The tympanometry showed low compliance on the right side, and left was inconclusive though it also showed diminished compliance with the possibility of middle ear effusion. PTA showed a moderate degree of high frequency sloping bilateral sensorineural hearing loss, which was slightly worse on the right side.

On functional testing, Mrs. P was unable to maintain her balance with reduced visual and proprioceptive inputs. Ocular-motor testing using VNG revealed no spontaneous, gaze evoked or rebound nystagmus. No abnormalities were detected upon testing of random saccades. Testing of smooth pursuit showed reduced velocity gain both on right and left side. Monothermal warm water caloric testing revealed a robust and approximately equal response bilaterally. Visual fixation index was normal.

It was therefore concluded the tests did not suggest any peripheral vestibular lesion. The moderately impaired pursuit may indicate a central lesion; however, the results may have been affected by her advanced age. It was felt that she may not benefit with vestibular exercises. Physiotherapy was, however, recommended, giving satisfactory response.

Five-Times-Sit-to-Stand Test is a relatively new entry in rehabilitation modalities for dizzy patients. Meretta et al. (2006) carried out a study to determine if patients with balance and vestibular disorders would demonstrate clinically meaningful improvement in the said test score as a result of vestibular rehabilitation and also to determine the concurrent validity of the FTSST.

It was a retrospective chart review of over 300 people who underwent individualised outpatient vestibular rehabilitation programmes in a tertiary balance clinic. Out of them, 117 patients with peripheral, central or mixed vestibular dysfunction in terms of FTSST, gait speed, Timed Up and Go Test (TUG), Dynamic Gait Index (DGI), Dizziness Handicap Inventory (DHI) and Activities-Specific Balance Confidence Scale (ABC) were investigated. Vestibular rehabilitation was moderately correlated with improvements in the DGI and the TUG scores ($p < 0.01$). This study confirmed that FTSST was responsive to change over time and was moderately related to measures of gait and dynamic balance.

The world grows increasingly older; therefore, more emphasis is being given to the care of the elderly, who suffer with many postural handicaps and have a strong tendency to fall. In a study (Macias et al. 2005), the efficacy of rehabilitation therapy was investigated. Short-term effectiveness of vestibular rehabilitation therapy in reducing fall risk in an at-risk population was measured. It was a retrospective chart review of 70 patients older than 50 years of age at risk for falls treated at a tertiary vestibular therapy centre. Fall risk was assessed by the Berg Balance Scale test. The authors noted that the vestibular rehabilitation therapy resulted in a statistically significant improvement in Berg Balance Scale test scores. Furthermore, they also noted that referring diagnosis, age and gender had no impact on outcome. Their conclusion was that vestibular rehabilitation therapy significantly reduces the risk of falls in at-risk elderly patients with improvement measured at the termination of therapy. It of course duly highlights the point that the vestibular rehabilitation therapy plays an important preventive role in reducing falls in at-risk elderly patients, with significant beneficial effects at the end of treatment.

Diabetes is known to cause many problems. It is characterised by the iconic triad of symptoms, namely, polyuria, polyphagia and polydipsia. Dizziness is one of the many symptoms of diabetes. Peripheral neuropathy is a known complication of uncontrolled diabetes. No wonder some older textbooks of medicine called it 'mother of all illnesses'.

In a study, the adverse effect of diabetic polyneuropathy was evaluated in vestibular disorders (Aranad et al. 2009). It was carried out to assess the influence of diabetic peripheral neuropathy on self-reported disability and postural control during quiet stance of patients with peripheral vestibular disease, before and after a standardised programme of vestibular rehab (Cawthorne and Cooksey) exercises. The study involved 27 patients. The observation made by the authors was that compared to the patients without neuropathy; those who had one, the neuropathy may indeed interfere with complete recovery. It appears that self-reported disability caused by neuropathy seems to contribute to the disability. In fact the picture gets quite confusing as one thing may lead to the other.

Drugs have always been used for the management of acute as well as chronic cases of vertigo. Vestibular rehabilitation therapy, however, has also stood the test of time in many cases.

Until recently most vertiginous patients were treated medically employing drugs like prochlorperazine, cinnarizine or betahistine, for indefinite periods of time. But a sea change has occurred in the management of vertigo, as the rehabilitation services have taken over the task with excellent outcomes.

We employ medical treatment in acute cases and rely heavily upon vestibular therapy; thus, a combination of both forms of treatment is currently in vogue in our hospitals as in many other centres.

Karapolat et al. (2010) investigated the hypothesis that a combined medicinal-rehab regime may have some additional benefits. They looked at the effect of high-dose betahistine treatment added to vestibular rehabilitation on disability as well as balance and postural stability in patients with unilateral vestibular disorder. After a comprehensive research, authors arrived at an affirmative result that betahistine added to VR was highly effective in managing these patients.

In the elderly population, reduced mobility markedly impairs quality of life, and the associated falls increase morbidity and mortality. Review of the literature based on a selective search and the findings of the authors' own studies on gait changes in old age and on the functional brain imaging of gait control was carried out. The study (Jahn et al. 2010) showed that gait disturbances in the elderly are often of multifactorial origin. The relevant pathogenic factors include sensory deficits such as visual, vestibular or somatosensory; neurodegenerative processes like cortical, extrapyramidal motor or cerebellar; and toxic factors such as those caused by drugs or alcohol; and anxiety or stress, or indeed the fear of falls. A clinically oriented classification of gait disorders is proposed by the authors. On the basis of the characterisation of gait and the accompanying clinical findings, it enables the identification of the etiological factors and points the way to rational therapy. The study concluded that the evaluation of elderly patients whose chief complaint is a gait disturbance should be directed towards the identification of specific deficits. This is the prerequisite for rational therapy, even when the problem is of multifactorial origin. The preservation of mobility is important in it and also because the ability to walk is closely correlated with cognitive performance.

We have good reasons to support this study, as we tend to differentiate between vertigo, which is a perception, and disequilibrium, which is a reality. The former can affect all age groups, the later mostly the elderly and otherwise moribund.

'Dizziness, vertigo, and imbalance are likely the most common presenting complaints among patients 75 years and older in office practices', thus observed by Ishiyama (2009). Although the cause of falls amongst the ageing population is multifactorial, several studies have implicated the peripheral vestibular organs. It is imperative that clinicians correctly diagnose and treat the vertigo in the geriatric population. Many studies have proven that vestibular impairment is quite responsive to specifically designed rehabilitation programmes. One of the commonest causes of vertigo in older adults is BPPV. The ageing otolith membrane, alterations in calcium metabolism and ischaemia have all been blamed as the possible factors. These authors also point out that age-related deterioration of vestibular function on quantitative testing has been documented. Besides, the age of onset correlates with the age-related cellular loss in the vestibular apparatus. According to these workers, it is likely that sensitivity of both the central and peripheral vestibular pathways plays a role in age-related decline in maintenance of posture.

Vestibular disorders in the older patients are associated with a diminished level of independent activities, an increased incidence of falls and masked or clinical depression. Co-morbidity is another matter that is a contributor in many elderly folks. The author's laboratory is delineating the immunohistochemical expression of proteins in the basement membrane of the vestibular system in the elderly as a potential cause of the age-related decline in sensory cell and neuronal population. Further tests and their results are keenly awaited. Once available, we should be able to understand the aetiopathogenesis even better.

It is generally agreed that for such patients as described by Ishiyama, conservative measures such as rehabilitation is the best form of management. It not only saves the patients from many an untold catastrophe, undue and unwanted long-term use of anti-vertiginous drugs but also alleviates their symptoms and improves their quality of life, considerably.

In our clinic, we often encounter the patients with a history of falls. Many of these patients end upon the emergency departments with broken bones or head injuries. In fact, a vast majority of these elderly patients are seen in the 'falls' clinic. Only some are referred to us for evaluation of vestibular system.

Many authors believed that vestibular rehabilitation therapy plays an important preventive role in reducing falls in at-risk elderly patients, with beneficial effects seen at termination of therapy. We concur with this study. Many of our elderly patients have shown major improvement in their quality of life as the fear of fall diminishes significantly with rehabilitation therapy. We believe that instead of treating these elderly folks with medicines alone, rehabilitation therapy alone or combined with drugs gives better and more satisfying results.

Ageing population has caused much concern to the physicians lately. Anxiety, stress, fear, psychological problems, etc. are common observations in the old patients. Compounded with those, if the patient has dizziness caused by vestibular pathology, the matter becomes even more challenging, both in diagnostic and in rehabilitative measures. Bou-Haidar et al. (2005) noted that vestibular abnormalities coexisting with anxiety disorders are not uncommon. There has been a renewal of interest in recent times on this subject. Although well known over centuries, there is often a delay in the recognition of this relationship by the primary care physician and the specialist alike. Dizziness, unsteadiness and imbalance are common in the elderly, so is the generalised anxiety disorder, a common psychiatric problem in later life. They investigated eight patients with dizziness, and anxiety disorder present with lack of awareness of their relationship was studied by these authors. The diagnoses of the anxiety disorders were based on the Diagnostic and Statistical Manual (DSM-IV) criteria. The effect of treatment was measured on a clinician-based impression interview. Apart from the vestibular symptoms present in all the patients, they also suffered with anxiety disorder, panic attacks and agoraphobia, hyperventilation, disturbed sleep, etc. They had all presented to the clinicians in different disciplines and had had several investigations carried out. Five had been treated in this study with alprazolam and three with citalopram, with modest to good results. Two of them received the rehabilitation therapy as well. The cases described mirror the well-documented coexistence of vestibular symptoms and anxiety disorders together with hyperventilation and sleep apnoea. Hyperventilation is often the only sign of masked anxiety and stress. Nijmegen scoring mentioned in this clinical guide is an invaluable tool for determining it. The positive findings associated with vestibular dysfunction need recognition in addition to the non-specific psychiatric and behavioural symptoms.

This study is an excellent pointer towards the fact that an elderly patient with imbalance may be seen with symptoms mentioned here, as the possible contributors to their co-morbidity.

China has an ancient history of medicine. From the prehistoric times, Chinese philosophy and their medical therapies have been documented in the world literature. Now that China is a superpower, much interest has grown into their ways of dealing with a multitude of problems, particularly through alternative therapies, albeit with guarded success.

Vestibular rehabilitation (VR) is a well-accepted practice intended to remedy balance impairment caused by damage to the peripheral vestibular system. One such exercise mentioned in the contemporary literature is that of Tai Chi (McGibbon et al. 2005).

The authors express that Tai Chi (TC) has recently gained popularity as a treatment for balance impairment. In fact, many doctors have taken it up as a routine morning exercise finding it comforting, soothing and relaxing.

Although vestibular rehabilitation and Tai Chi can benefit people with vestibulopathy, the degree to which gait improvements may be related to neuromuscular adaptations of the lower extremities for the two different therapies is unknown. We have a few patients who have benefitted with Tai Chi and simply love going to these sessions, finding them extremely helpful in bringing back their daily activities to their satisfaction. Obviously we as clinicians are not fully aware of the mode of action of such therapies, as some similar treatments may have a placebo rather than a therapeutic effect, but it seems to work in some and is harmless, noninvasive and fun. One particular woman of 82 claimed that no one could help her regain her balance, but the Tai Chi master did!

Nevertheless, the study concluded that gait function improved in both groups consistent with expectations of the interventions. Differences in each group's response to therapy appear to suggest that improved gait function may be due to different neuromuscular adaptations resulting from the different interventions. The TC group's improvements were associated with reorganised lower-extremity neuromuscular patterns, which appear to promote a faster gait and reduced excessive hip compensation. The VR group's improvements, however, were not the result of lower-extremity neuromuscular pattern changes. Lower-extremity MEE increases corresponded to attenuated forward trunk linear and angular movement in the VR group, suggesting better control of upper body motion to minimise loss of balance. These authors believe that due to a growing body of evidence, Tai Chi may be a valuable complementary treatment for vestibular disorders.

Cohen and Kimball (2004) investigated the effects of vestibular rehabilitation on gait, ataxia and balance. The patients with chronic vertigo due to peripheral vestibular impairments were investigated. They were assessed on the Timed Up and Go

Test, ataxia during a path integration test, Computerised Dynamic Posturography, level of vertigo, independence in activities of daily living and psychological locus of control. They were randomly assigned to three home programme treatment groups. It was a useful and time-consuming but comprehensive study. After an exhaustive research, it was thus concluded that the ataxia decreased significantly, and posturography scores and time to perform Timed Up and Go improved significantly, for all subjects. Improvements were significantly related to scores on the ambulation subtest of the Vestibular Disorders Activities of Daily Living Scale, decrease in vertigo and increase in locus of control. It was concluded by the authors that for many patients, a simple home programme of vestibular habituation head movement exercises is related to reduce symptoms of imbalance during stance and gait.

One major problem encountered in clinical practice is that of investigating and managing a case of unilateral vestibular dysfunction.

Topuz and colleagues (2004) measured the efficacy of vestibular rehabilitation exercises on patients with chronic unilateral vestibular dysfunction in over a 100 patients. It was a fairly large sample of cohorts. The study demonstrated that a fast recovery was noticed in the supervised exercise session, whereas no significant difference was seen in the domestic setting. These findings suggested that supervised exercise was better than housebound exercise. The proponents of this study also advocated that a few supervised sessions were sufficient to obtain the desirable result. The relevance of the study is particularly important in these days of emphasis on managing the patients at home and in their own surroundings rather than treating them in rehab centres.

Another study by Badke et al. (2004) involved evaluation of outcomes after vestibular rehabilitation in adult population, namely, the balance, dynamic gait and dynamic visual acuity. It was also designed to determine certain variables significantly associated with improved balance and ambulation. It was a brief study on only 20 cohorts, managed for about 11 months. One might criticise this study on the basis of a small sample size, but its validity cannot be denied. The only criticism could be on the improvement of visual acuity that the authors claim to have improved with therapy. Obviously one would expect an improvement due to correction of refraction or perhaps a surgical intervention such as a lens replacement and not just the physical therapy as appears to be the case here.

Anyhow, this study showed that the patients showed functional improvements in balance, visual acuity and gait stability after vestibular physical therapy. Age and pre-therapy vertical dynamic visual acuity score influenced dynamic gait outcome after a balance rehabilitation programme. These parameters are best known to our colleagues in the rehab services as they can gauge them more efficiently than the clinicians. The clinical measurement is based upon a history of increased physical activity, going out and about and taking care of personal chores. Such parameters need basic interrogation regarding the daily activities.

We tend not to think of vestibular pathology confined to only one ear, though it is a fairly common finding. Unilateral vestibular dysfunction was, therefore, the subject of another study by Schubert et al. (2004), a few years ago.

It was designed to determine whether the cervico-ocular reflex contributed to gaze stability in such patients. The study involved patients before and after vestibular rehabilitation, and seven healthy subjects were taken as a control.

The authors found no evidence of cervico-ocular reflex in any of the seven healthy subjects as well as in two of the patients with unilateral vestibular hypofunction. In one patient with chronic unilateral vestibular hypofunction, the cervico-ocular reflex was present before vestibular rehabilitation only for leftward trunk rotation. After 5 weeks of placebo exercises, there was no change in the cervico-ocular reflex. After an additional 5 weeks that included vestibular exercises, cervico-ocular reflex gain for leftward trunk rotation had increased threefold. In addition, they also noticed some evidence of a cervico-ocular reflex for rightward trunk rotation, potentially compensating for the vestibular deficit. It was therefore concluded that the cervico-ocular reflex appeared to be a highly inconsistent mechanism. The change of the cervico-ocular reflex in one patient after vestibular exercises suggested that this reflex may indeed be adaptable in some patients. Suffice it to say that such research studies as this one provide new opportunities for us to explore further the many intricate mechanisms and sensitive pointers related to posture control.

As mentioned before, many dizzy patients present with a recent or a past history of falls. Many times, they do not even mention it unless specifically probed.

Edelberg (2003) believes that most falls result from the accumulated effect of multiple disease-related or intrinsic and environment-related or extrinsic factors. Falls often serve as non-specific markers of underlying disease and disability in older adults and may be the first sign of an acute illness or an exacerbation of a chronic illness. In this paper, he also includes the recommendations for therapeutic and preventive approaches to non-syncopal fall, which are characterised by a transient loss of consciousness and spontaneous recovery. The goals of care are to minimise the risk of falls without compromising mobility or functional independence and also to prevent relevant fall-related morbidities such as bony injuries, fear of fall and the inability to get up, after a fall.

Traditionally Cawthorne–Cooksey exercises have been the pillar of strength for the rehabilitation teams since the past four or five decades. They have stood the test of time, in the commoner variety of bilateral vestibular disorders. Unilateral vestibulopathy is relatively less of a problem. But it can be.

Corma et al. (2003) carried out a study to evaluate the efficiency of these rehab exercises in unilateral vestibular disorders. It was carried out at the division of physical therapy and rehabilitation at a scientific institute in Italy. They inferred that both the Cawthorne–Cooksey and instrumental rehabilitation were effective for treating vestibular vertigo. Improvement of the control of body balance and performance of daily activities was a major benefit achieved. They believed that the larger decrease in body sway and greater improvement of daily activities after instrumental rehabilitation made them favour over Cawthorne–Cooksey exercises in improving the postural control.

Most cases dealt with by the ENT specialists are of peripheral vestibular origin. We know there are many central pathologies known to cause vertigo. Their rehabilitation is always more demanding and challenging with limited outcomes. Suarez et al. (2003) looked at the postural responses before and after a vestibular rehabilitation in patients with central vestibular disorders. After a comprehensive evaluation, it was concluded from the study that many of these patients damaged the neural mechanisms involved in retaining the plastic changes in the postural control after rehabilitative treatment. The authors advised long-term training protocol, to maintain the improvement obtained with initial vestibular rehabilitation therapy.

Vestibular rehabilitation has proved to be an extremely potent tool in managing patients with vertigo. Cohen and Kimball (2003) sought out to determine just that, if vestibular rehabilitation was indeed effective in decreasing the vertigo, and increasing performance of daily life skills in the patients of peripheral vestibular lesions were seen at a tertiary care centre. They were assessed on the basis of the intensity and frequency of dizziness, employing various tools of measurement such as the following: the Vertigo Symptom Scale, the Vertigo Handicap Questionnaire, the Vestibular Disorders Activities of Daily Living Scale and the Dizziness Handicap Inventory.

The results showed that vertigo decreased and independence in activities of daily living improved significantly. Variables like age, gender or the history of vertigo had no direct bearing on the results.

It was noted at the end of the study that for many patients, a simple home programme of vestibular habituation and head movement exercises led to reduction in symptoms thereby increasing independence in daily activities. And no one can argue with the point that independence is an invaluable attribute to possess in this age group as indeed in most.

Driving with dizziness is a dangerous business. Most physicians would warn the patients if not altogether stop them from driving.

Cohen and Kimball (2003) believe that there are few studies that have queried the patients about their driving performance: so the data is insufficient. They designed a Driving Habits Questionnaire and conducted structured interviews with people with several different vestibular disorders employing normal subjects as control. The self-reported crash rate and rate of citations for moving violations did not differ between the subject groups. Interesting results were noted in this study. Patients report reduced driving skills, particularly in situations when visual information is reduced, rapid head movements are used, and specific path integration or spatial navigation skills are needed.

The move towards evidence-based practice has encouraged clinicians to re-evaluate the evidence for many established therapies (Gee and Humphriss 2003).

Vestibular rehabilitation is a popular treatment for patients with motion sickness and has received growing interest in the UK over the last 10 years. This chapter applies the principle of evidence-based medicine to published studies on rehab therapy. Although a shortage of randomised controlled trials about vestibular rehabilitation has been identified, the literature in general concludes that it is an effective treatment for many diagnostic categories of balance disorder patient. There is a need for more of randomised controlled trials to be carried out in the future in order to establish the true efficacy of this treatment.

Age-related dizziness is a major issue these days. Besides, compared with younger subjects, many such cases do not show such a good response with rehabilitation therapy. It is a slightly debatable issue though, as the will to fight has a lot to do with the rehab therapy as well as the will to live freely and independently. Some older folks, therefore, do better than others. The following study by Whitney et al. (2002) prove the point that age may not have much influence on the final outcome of rehabilitation therapy though some clinicians may not agree with their observations.

The purpose of the retrospective chart review was to compare vestibular rehabilitation outcomes in young versus older adults. Twenty-three persons with vestibular disorders aged 20–40 years were matched by gender, vestibular diagnosis and vestibular function test results to 23 older adults aged 60–80 years. Younger adults had more impaired DGI scores and a higher proportion of caloric testing abnormalities. After rehabilitation, overall improvement was seen in both the younger and older populations. There were no statistical differences between the two groups on the DHI, the DGI, reported symptoms at discharge and number of falls. When only the complete matched-pair data were analysed, there were no statistically significant differences between the age groups in the proportion of patients demonstrating clinical improvement. It was observed by these authors that age does not significantly influence the beneficial effects of vestibular rehabilitation for persons with vestibular disorders.

Disequilibrium or imbalance is indeed a major problem to solve. It affects all age groups and is often associated with co-morbidity in the form of physical, social, psychological and financial resources. Much research goes on in the world to tackle the issue more effectively. The diagnosis of imbalance has become somewhat simpler with the addition of modern tools described in this book. Management, however, continues to pose a formidable challenge. Rehabilitation is one invaluable way of managing such patients.

Several studies are quoted here which duly support the evidence that in most peripheral vestibular and many central conditions leading to vertigo, vestibular rehabilitation is an extremely useful, helpful and a valuable tool.

References

Aranad C, Meza A, Rodriguez R, Mantilla MT, Jaureui-Renaud K (2009) Diabetic poly neuropathy may increase the handicap related to vestibular disease. Arch Med Res 40(3):180–185

Badke MB, Shea TA, Miedaner JA, Grove CR (2004) Outcomes after rehabilitation for adults with balance dysfunction. Arch Phys Med Rehabil 85(2):227–233

Childs LA (2010) Assessing vestibular dysfunction. Exploring treatments of a complex condition. Rehab Manag 23(6):0899–6237, 0899–6237

Cohen HS, Kimball KT (2003) Increased independence and decreased vertigo after vestibular rehabilitation. Otolaryngol Head Neck Surg 128(1):60–70

Cohen HS, Kimball KT (2004) Decreased ataxia and improved balance after vestibular rehabilitation. Otolaryngol Head Neck Surg 130(4):418–425, 0194–5998

Corna S, Nardone A, Prestinari A, Galante M, Grasso M, Schieppati M (2003) Comparison of Cawthorne-Cooksey exercises and sinusoidal support surface translations to improve balance in patients with unilateral vestibular deficit. Arch Phys Med Rehabil 84(8):1173–1184

Edelberg HK (2003) Evaluation and management of fall risk in the older adults. Annals of Long-Term Care 11(10):34–40, 1524–7929 (Oct 2003)

Gee RD, Humphriss RL (2003) What is the evidence base for vestibular rehabilitation? CME Bull Otorhinolaryngol Head Neck Surg 7(2):35–37

Ischiyama G (2009) Imbalance and vertigo: the ageing human vestibular periphery. Semin Neurol 29(5):491–499, 0271–8235; 1098–9021. (Nov 2009)

Jahn K, Zwergal A, Schniepp R (2010) Gait disturbances Classification, diagnosis, and treatment from a neurological perspectiveGangstorungen im alter – Klassifikation, diagnostik und therapie aus neurologischer sicht. Dtsch Arztebl Int 107(17):306–316, 0012–1207 (30 Apr 2010

Karapolat H, Celebisoy N, Kirazli Y, Bilgen C, Eyigor S, Gode S, Akyuz A, Kirazli T (2010) Does betahistine treatment have additional benefits to vestibular rehabilitation? Eur Arch Otorhinolaryngol 267(8):1207–1212, 0937–4477 (August 2010)

Macias JD, Massingale S, Gerkin RD (2005) Efficacy of vestibular rehabilitation therapy in reducing falls. Otolaryngol Head Neck Surg 133(3):323–325, 0194–5998; 0194–5998 (2005 Sep)

McGibbon CA, Krebs DE, Parker SW, Scarborough DM, Wayne PM, Wolf SL (2005) Tai Chi and vestibular rehabilitation improve vestibulopathy gait via different neuromuscular mechanisms: preliminary report. BMC Neurol 5(1):3, 1471–2377; 1471–2377 (2005 Feb 18)

Meretta BM, Whitney SL, Marchetti GF, Sparto PJ, Muirhead RJ (2006) The five times sit to stand test: responsiveness to change and concurrent validity in adults undergoing vestibular rehabilitation. J Vestib Res 16(4–5):233–243, 0957–4271; 0957–4271

Nagaratnam N, Ip J, Bou-Haidar P (2005) The vestibular dysfunction and anxiety disorder interface: a descriptive study with special reference to the elderly. Arch Gerontol Geriatr 40(3):253–264, 0167

Polat S, Polat S, Uneri A (2010) Vestibular substitution:a comparative study. J Laryngol Otol 124(8):852–858, 0022–2151; 1748–5460

Schubert MC, Das V, Tusa RJ, Herdman SJ (2004) Cervico-ocular reflex in normal subjects and patients with unilateral vestibular hypo function. Otol Neurotol 25(1):65–71, 1531–7129; 1531–7129 (2004)

Suarez H, Arocena M, Suarez A, De Artagaveytia TA, Muse P, Gil J (2003) Postural control parameters after vestibular rehabilitation in changes in patients with central vestibular disorders. Acta Otolaryngol 123(2):143–147, 0001–6489; 0001–6489

Topuz O, Topuz B, Ardic FN, Sarhus M, Ogmen G, Ardic F (2004) Efficacy of vestibular rehabilitation on chronic unilateral vestibular dysfunction. Clin Rehabil 18(1):76–83, 0269–2155 (Feb 2004)

Virk S, McConville KM (2006) Virtual reality applications in improving postural control and minimizing falls. Conf Proc IEEE Eng Med Biol Soc 1:2694–2697, 1557–170X; 1557–170X (2006)

Whitney SL, Wrisley DM, Marchetti GF, Furman JM (2002) The effect of age on vestibular rehabilitation outcomes. Laryngoscope 112(10):1785–1790, 0023–852X; 0023–852X (2002Oct) 0194–5998; 0194–5998 (2003 Jan)

Vertigo in the Elderly: Quality of Life and Some Ethical Issues

12

Medicine without medical ethics is akin to a mother without motherhood. Both are intertwined and quite inseparable from times immemorial. Rapid advances in health care and longevity of life have cropped up many a fresh dilemma for the physician. Dealing with children, minors and handicapped is another issue, which is causing much concern to the health authorities. The recent exposé of a television celebrity's affair in the UK has all but destroyed the faith of an ordinary citizen in the people who matter. Surely there are many untold stories related to the abuse of children and the elderly that remain under the dark corridors of human conscience. The elderly suffer humiliation and indignity by the carers and the mentally retrace at the hands of inhuman caretakers all the time.

Morality is an inborn element. It is not necessary to be a believer to be moral, nor is it true that a nonbeliever would always be an amoral person. It is a trait that one is born with, though duly cultivated by the family through their practices, values, norms and principles. Medicine demands that one must be ethical and moral in dealing with fellow human beings. The fundamental principles of bioethics are autonomy, beneficence, non-maleficence and justice. They must all be followed with honesty and integrity.

WHO and the savants in the field of health economics have coined some highly meaningful catch phrases over the last couple of decades. One such term is the impact of disease on human health or more specifically called the 'Global Burden of Disease on Health (GBD)'. It has many nuances and ramifications in a person's working life as indeed on the community in general. No doubt vertigo is such a clinical condition that causes significant morbidity and incapacity to the sufferers, resulting in loss of work thus economic burden on the people's family and the society as result thereof.

Another interesting terminology used is QALY or quality-adjusted life years. It has a very complex mathematical formula that the health economists employ to reach a decision as to whether a given condition and a given treatment would result in x number of quality-adjusted life years or not. It is seldom if at all applicable to ordinary cases of benign vertigo but may be considered in certain central conditions causing incurable vertigo.

S.H. Zaidi, A. Sinha, *Vertigo*,
DOI 10.1007/978-3-642-36485-3_12, © Springer-Verlag Berlin Heidelberg 2013

QALY has been defined as a measure of burden of diseases on the society/community/humanity both in quantitative as well as qualitative terms. It is used by health economists and the 'gate keepers' as a tool for measurement of the values for money for a medical intervention. It is calculated on the basis of number of years of life that would be added upon a given intervention. The value given to a year in life is 1 and to death 0. So, for example, if patient loses a part of his body, an organ, an eye or limb and cannot maintain a normal healthy life without wheelchair support, then the extra life years are calculated between 0 and 1 to account for it. It is a measure of cost-utility designed to calculate the ratio of cost to QALYs saved for particular intervention. It is then used as parameter to decide the distribution of health resources. Rationing in today's health-care system has become a norm; hence, all the debate that goes on in the media as to who, when and why should one get preference over another patient if everyone is contributing equally to the service. This utilitarian approach in today's health care is often condemned by many ethicists who are strong proponents of Deontology.

The tools employed for QALYS are time trade-off, standard gamble and visual analogue scale. Further details can be obtained in the journals of medical ethics.

Quality of life is currently an important parameter that seems to interest the health economists and, truly enough, it has a major role to play in one's life. A patient suffering with Meniere's may find it hard to go out and about without the fear of facing another spontaneous bouts of dizziness, even a fall, resulting in a head or limb injury. Perhaps QALY would be more applicable in those intractable or incurable cases of vertigo such as an acoustic neuroma in a patient requiring labyrinthectomy, etc. than ordinary cases of vertigo. Nevertheless, it is a measure that determines the application and outcome of a given health service and distribution of resources depending on their availability.

According to Yardley et al. (2003), vertigo is often reported to be the most distressing aspect of having Meniere's disease and is the symptom that has the greatest impact on life. Many such patients do indeed say exactly that. They are afraid to go out shopping on their own or visit a public place as they have a fear lurking in their psyche of developing an acute attack like they 'once' had: which may incapacitate them for awhile.

Vertigo does not only have a physiological impact but also physical and psychological. One volatile episode of acute fulminating labyrinthitis may shake up an elderly woman's confidence so much that later on even a slight sensation of momentary light-headedness may result in her reaching for the bed, thus compromising her quality of life. A severe bout of Meniere's disease may be as traumatic psychologically as having a heart attack, resulting in similar prevalence levels of a condition called post-traumatic stress disorder. Describing the psychological aspects of Meniere's disease, Kirby and Yardley (2008) have discussed three main groups of symptoms in post-traumatic stress disorder. The first includes a sense of re-experiencing the event through invasive memories, thoughts, etc. The second group of symptoms include avoiding or being unable to recall activities, people or places that may bring back bad memories of the vertiginous attack. The third group of symptoms include feeling emotionally numb or detached from others (Kirby and Yardley 2009).

Further details of their interesting observations may be obtained through their original publication in the ENT news last year.

The microanatomy, neurophysiology of PTSD and neurochemical factors underlying the mechanics of PTSD has been investigated by some experts. Of all the structures in the CNS, it appears that amygdala is most directly implicated in the evaluation of the emotional meaning of incoming stimuli. Amygdala, as we know, has extensive connections within the cortical neurogenic tissue. Charney et al. (1993) suggest the possibility that many memories associated with traumatic events will be ultimately stored in the cortex. They believe that amygdala may play a crucial role in the ability of specific sensory stimuli to elicit traumatic memories. Fear is an essential aspect of vertiginous conditions as indeed many other psychophysiological diseases. According to LeDoux, thalamo-amygdala connections provide rapid reactions to fear-conditioned stimuli, while thalamo-cortico-amygdala circuits may act relatively slowly and possibly subserve more elaborated kinds of fear (LeDoux 1992).

In stressful conditions, the sympathetic nervous system becomes active resulting in activation of the adrenal gland, releasing epinephrine, norepinephrine and steroidal hormones. It is this physiological act that enables us to stand firm and harness our residual resources to combat an unusual or a stressful situation. Sports persons thrive upon it.

Hassan et al. (1999) discussed the subject of psychobiology of post-traumatic stress disorder. It is a common practice to see the patients of vertigo suffering with loneliness, depression, anxiety, emotional stress and lack of physical activity. It is the perpetual fear of facing another attack that seems to trigger off the initial fear which then takes the shape and form a vicious cycle. They have a tendency to give up work, which means going on benefits, yet other sources of burden on society, loneliness due to loss of social activity, lack of communication resulting in solitude and finally tendency to curl up in a cocoon of depression, hopelessness and misery.

It is absolutely vital that taking up such jobs that may potentiate vertigo must be avoided. For instance, a roof layer with a history of Meniere's will be ill advised to climb the roof to lay a roof. Likewise, a machinist working on a sawmill or in a foundry with extremely hot iron pouring out, or the machine revolving at the speed of a space shuttle, may not work in this kind of environment. As a matter of fact, even the non-suspecting person who has a fear of heights may not be encouraged to climb a fast-moving lift or go on a joy ride in a theme park that may stimulate his labyrinth possessing a low threshold.

Many patients would restrict their physical activity to avoid precipitation of vertigo. It has been described as 'anticipatory disability' (Cioffi 1991). It has sometimes been ascribed to a fearful or passive mode of responding to physical ailments (Yardley 1994). Such a limitation of activity is self-defeating indeed. The fear of movement potentiating an acute attack of vertigo is perceptual rather than sporadic and pathological. It has to have an underlying diseased vestibular system to bring about vertigo, as a healthy system should not and will not bring about vertigo on simple physical movements. And that is where it is absolutely vital that the patients' self-confidence should be built to face the reality and not live in a world of apprehension, fear and self-imposed intimidation. Psychologists inform us that the role of an ENT/vestibular team remains incomplete and the job unfulfilled if the underlying fear of motion triggering off vertigo is not duly resolved.

This is exactly what the patients feel. They are literally housebound for the apprehension feeling that going out and about may make them sick, and the jolts faced by any bus traveller seem to worry them a great deal. They are always concerned about a fall; hence, they find it hard to carry out their daily chores resulting in untidiness and neglected personal hygiene.

Many patients find it difficult to understand that the attack of Meniere's may not always come about at regular intervals. And because in Meniere's there are natural periods of remission, initially they find it hard to believe that the problem may have been only temporarily halted and that another attack may not appear for several months, even years. The confidence that shakes up with the first attack is extremely difficult to build up.

As mentioned elsewhere in this book, one reason why such patients should not be given long-term labyrinthine sedatives is that the normal vestibular compensatory action would inevitably be delayed leading to drug dependence. This practice must be discouraged and only a minimum course of labyrinthine sedatives be given.

The fear of heights or acrophobia is a known entity. In patients suffering from vertigo due to an underlying vestibular disorder, the susceptibility to vertical heights as well as horizontal motion sickness seems to become more pronounced. It is therefore obvious that they must be warned against such leisure activities as climbing the mountains or driving a racing car or a high or fast-moving swing or a ride in a theme park.

Many patients with chronic vertigo become so lazy that they put on excessive weight, resulting in many secondary problems. It is a common observation that these patients often complain of lower backache and neck stiffness. It is true, though some people argue against it, that cervical osteoarthritis seems to potentiate vertigo. The fear of moving the neck about causes further stiffening of the neck resulting in more discomfort particularly at level of the root of the neck.

Assurance is vital. The neck movement must be continued or else the stiffness by itself may aggravate aches and pains in the upper body. The restriction of neck movement with the application of a cervical collar was a common practice a couple of decades ago. It has been totally replaced with appropriate physiotherapy and suitable neck and upper torso exercises to improve the physiological function of the neck muscles. The proprioceptive impulses going from the neck receptors play a pivotal role in maintenance of balance.

Driving is another important issue. No doubt a person who has repeated bouts of vertigo is not only a potential risk to himself but indeed to the public at large. He is therefore best advised to avoid driving and inform the DVLA or the relevant licensing authority, about his driving status. They have their medical department that shall advise the patient after careful consideration of the history and clinical diagnosis.

Once the acute stage is over and his compensatory mechanisms have taken over, he may be able to drive under caution. Patients with Meniere's disease are known to experience an aura before an impending attack. They are therefore self-disciplined and do not drive or indeed perform any such act that may endanger their life or of those in the neighbourhood.

The burden of disease and disability is borne by the taxpayer in most countries. In many other countries, which lack the social services, this burden is happily shared by the family. Anthropologists inform us that in the Asian communities and many Far Eastern countries, it is a norm to have large families sharing home and hearth. In the Chinese communities too, this phenomenon is witnessed not just in their homeland but all over the world wherever they may live. It is all a matter of cultural norms. Altruism is a universal practice, which is perhaps more visible in the Asian culture.

The impact of culture on mental and psychological health is a very established and highly debated subject. There are certain specific culture or culture-specific psychiatric syndromes such as koro and latah Silva de Pdamal (1999).

The term culture has been defined by sociologists and anthropologists in many ways. It may mean different things to different people. It includes values, norms, practices, faith, beliefs, habits, family pattern, upbringing, taboos, sanctions and dietary habits.

It is a common observation that in many developing nations, the family bondage is so strong that the burden of the disease and disability does not affect the society as it does in the developed nations. It is, however, a rapidly receding trait.

Post-traumatic stress disorder is a relatively new diagnostic category but carries enormous significance in describing or managing the impact of a traumatic condition on a human being. Yardley has written extensively on the subject which is mentioned in this book elsewhere. Although some famous politicians of recent times denied the existence of 'society' in their political speeches, most sociologists would disagree and stress that the society or a community is indeed a collection of many individuals. Therefore, it is illogical to assume that the impact of traumatic situation affecting an individual may indeed be reflected in the collective response of the community. In the bygone days when mankind lived in the forests and had to hunt for his meal, tribal culture developed in response to the collective needs of time such as protection and safety. Even today in many parts of the developing countries, a tribal head, who is usually an unkind person, is more revered than the king emperor, and the tribal customs are more valuable than any legal or religious commandment. History informs us that even though the prophets, savants and the saviours came to serve the divine commands, but more often than not, they had to accept and imbibe the cultural norms of the society and only gradually if at all discard them over a period of time.

The dizzy elderly patient with a cardiovascular or a central disorder or indeed a relapsing vestibular disease in a family setting does not feel isolated or depressed. The same cannot be said of the modern families where the family is no more than just a couple and many times not even that, as single parenthood is becoming increasingly common. Therefore, a dizzy patient has to be referred for care to the social workers or the institutions depending upon the nature and intensity of the problem.

Old age is often associated with gait disturbances as indeed with the repeated episodes of falls. Partly it is due to genuine physico-pathological reasons, but partly it is also the fear of fall and apprehension to walk unsupported that the elderly find it hard to go out and about.

In an excellent study at Duke (Slaone et al. 1989), many factors were identified to contribute to the disequilibrium of old age. It was noted that some of these elderly folks may suffer from a 'syndrome of multiple neurosensory deficits'. This may result from deficient functioning of some of the sensory systems that help regulate equilibrium. They are vestibular, ocular, cervical proprioceptive, central vestibular, cerebellar and peripheral sensory systems.

This study also identified two groups of elderly patients presenting with dizziness. The larger of the two groups comprised of people with anxiety, depression and other psychosomatic ailments. The second category consisted of patients of CVS, metabolic, neurosensory and drug-related problems.

Many of our patients fall into both these categories, though in some, one can never identify the primary reason, as a multifactorial clinical entity may indeed have multiple underlying factors albeit with one common presentation.

Case Report

P was born in March 1930s and presented with spells of rotatory vertigo with associated nausea about 15 years ago. She described being unable to walk in a straight line and had to remain in bed for a few days feeling unwell for a period of about 2–3 weeks. Her hearing apparently deteriorated for 2–3 days, and she felt that sounds felt distorted when the hearing returned initially. She said that her hearing loss in the left ear began at that time. She also described having undergone tests for her dizziness, which sounded like calorimetry; following which, she was told that she suffered with Meniere's disease.

Mrs. P said that she did not experience any rotatory vertigo or be bedridden since her initial attack 15 years ago. She, however, said that she used to experience spells of imbalance two or three times a year. She was prescribed SERC, which she stopped taking about 6 years ago. Since then, she took a diuretic tablet and felt symptom-free for the last 4–5 years until the August/ September of 2009. At this time, she felt off balance and almost as if drunk, upon waking up in the morning. The feeling lasted for 3 days. She also noticed a reduction in her hearing lasting a day followed by distortion of sounds. In between the attacks, Mrs. P experienced light-headedness on bending down and upon standing up. She reported that 2 years ago, she had turned her head quickly which had led to her fall. She said that she is currently leading a normal life and doing her daily chores without a problem.

Mrs. P denied tinnitus, though she noticed a feeling of constant pressure in her left ear without noticing any change in this feeling during the spells of imbalance. Mrs. P also told that she had a mastoid operation done upon her as a baby (which could have been a drainage of an abscess or a cortical mastoidectomy, though the scar was imperceptible on inspection).

Mrs. P also suffered with migraines as a teenager causing her severe headaches and dizziness. She also had sustained an attack of angina 30 years ago and suffered with hypothyroidism. Therefore, she was on thyroxin, a benzoflouride and a beta blocker. Mrs. P also has cervical arthritis without causing any noticeable restriction of her neck movements.

Otoscopy revealed no abnormalities. The tympanometry indicated normal middle ear function bilaterally. Pure tone audiometry showed a moderate degree of sensorineural hearing loss confined to the higher frequencies in the right ear and a similar loss involving all the frequencies on the left side. Slight improvement was noted at 250 K on the left side compared to an audiogram recorded 4 months earlier.

On functional testing, Mrs. P was unable to maintain her balance with reduced visual and proprioceptive inputs. Ocular-motor testing using VNG revealed no spontaneous or rebound nystagmus. Upon gaze testing without fixation, a low-level right beating nystagmus was noticed, with eyes directed to the right, and a low-level left beating nystagmus with eyes directed to the left. This may, however, have been an end point nystagmus as she had difficulty keeping her eyes in the correct position. Testing of random saccades and smooth pursuit showed no abnormalities. Calorimetry was not undertaken due to her unsettled angina.

The results of vestibular tests, therefore, did not suggest any central or peripheral vestibular lesion. Calorimetry would have been of immense help but was contraindicated. Elements of her history and the slight change in her hearing on the left side were in keeping with Meniere's disease, which was diagnosed in her many years ago when she apparently had undergone calorimetry also.

She was advised to return to the outpatient clinic for a follow-up.

Case Report

Mrs. P was born in the early 1940s and was seen in our vestibular lab for detailed assessment in April 2010. She reported two episodes of recent bouts of dizziness, which she described as rotatory in nature initiated by her turning her head in bed. It lasted for less than a minute and was followed by disequilibrium and imbalance for about an hour. She also reported the onset of similar, more marked, symptoms in January 2010, when undergoing exercises given by her GP that involved head turns. There was no associated nausea during the previous episodes. She, however, said that she had sensation of 'heaviness' in her left ear, a reduction in hearing in her left ear and an exacerbation of her long-standing left-sided tinnitus. In the week leading up to the episodes of dizziness at least on two previous occasion in September 2009 and January 2010. She mentioned that gaze fixation helped to alleviate her symptoms during a spell, and she had a tendency to guard against getting out of bed too quickly for the fear of provoking her symptoms, although it had been less frequent since November.

Mrs. P also reported an episode of rotatory vertigo in 1997; the symptoms of which lasted half away and caused her to stagger when she tried to walk. She said she was unwell at the time and had no associated nausea or variation in her hearing or indeed tinnitus. She, however, noticed heaviness in her left ear during the spell but said that she also had trigeminal neuralgia at the time, though it was diagnosed a few years later, in 2005.

Mrs. P reported a fluctuating, left-sided gradual deterioration in her hearing over the last 3–4 years. She also reported a continuous 'buzzing' left-sided tinnitus, more pronounced when she also noticed a decline in her hearing. She also noticed increased heaviness in her left ear at that time. She also received medication for her coronary heart disease.

The otoscopy examination was normal bilaterally. Tympanometry was fine on each side too, with ipsilateral acoustic reflexes showing normal recordings on each side. Pure tone audiometry showed normal hearing levels on the right side with the exception of 25 dbHL threshold at 8 kHZ and a mild sensorineural hearing loss on the left side. Deterioration in hearing thresholds was noted compared with the tests recorded in March 2008.

Upon functional testing, Mrs. P was able to maintain her balance with reduced visual and proprioceptive inputs. Oculomotor testing using VNG revealed no spontaneous, gaze-evoked or rebound nystagmus. No abnormalities were detected upon testing of random saccades or smooth pursuit. Dix–Hallpike testing was negative bilaterally. Monothermal screening caloric test using warm water produced robust and approximately equal responses bilaterally. Visual fixation index was normal.

It was therefore inferred that Mrs. P had Meniere's disease with possibility of fluctuating vestibular functions. It was also considered a possibility that Mrs. P also had suffered with BPPV which had resolved spontaneously.

Case Report

Mr. P was born in 1941 and presented with a history of an ear infection in his right ear a year ago followed by imbalance until now. He also noticed lightheadedness on standing up from a sitting posture or indeed on moving around. He felt that he may fall down while walking up the stairs.

No abnormalities were noted on otoscopy with normal tympanometry bilaterally. Ocular-motor testing revealed no significant spontaneous, gaze-evoked or rebound nystagmus. No abnormalities of saccadic eye movements were detected either. Mr. P continually jumped his eyes on smooth pursuit;

this may have been due to failure to fully comprehend the test and its motives. Conventional calorimetry revealed a significant canal paresis on the right side, with marked directional preponderance to the left.

It was therefore concluded from the results that a significant peripheral vestibular weakness existed on the right side. Poor smooth pursuit could well be a central sign but can also be caused by lack of attention or failure to concentrate. Mr. S was advised to commence Cawthorne–Cooksey exercise with a follow-up appointment to monitor his progress.

Case Report

P, born in late 1970s, was seen in the vestibular lab in February 2010, with a history of imbalance for the last 3 months. She described her symptoms to appear spontaneously in the middle of the night with a sensation of vertigo and vomiting. The sensation continued for a couple of weeks. It then reduced to daily spells noticed upon movement only and further reduced to similar episodes noticed only four to five times in a week. She describes her 'feeling akin' to 'standing on water'. It could be provoked by rapid head movement, bending forward and brisk postural changes. She also felt a falling sensation on lying on her right side in the bed.

Mrs. P wore hearing aids bilaterally and said that her hearing loss began about 18 months ago had deteriorated gradually over the last few months. She had no familial history of deafness or hearing impairment and suffered with occasional tinnitus worse on the right side. Neither the hearing loss nor tinnitus fluctuated with dizziness. She had frequent headaches, along with migraine and visual disturbances. Ms. P also suffered from asthma, fibromyalgia and epilepsy and had Ehlers–Danlos syndrome.

No abnormalities were noted on otoscopy. PTA indicated a severe bilateral hearing loss, which was mixed in nature in at least one ear. Tympanometry was bilaterally normal.

Ocular-motor testing using videonystagmography revealed no spontaneous, rebound or gaze-evoked nystagmus. No abnormalities of smooth pursuit were detected. Saccadic eye movements had prolonged latency in both right and left directions. Accuracy and velocity of saccade was within the normal limits to the left, but borderline to the right. The Dix–Hallpike testing was negative bilaterally. Calorimetry was contraindicated on account of her epilepsy. The handshake test provoked a right beating nystagmus. The head thrust test was bilaterally negative.

It was therefore concluded that a peripheral vestibular lesion affecting the left ear was a strong possibility. The abnormal saccades may suggest a central lesion; however, 'normal range' of saccadic parameters is thought to be different in epileptic patients.

Ms. P was commenced on Cawthorne–Cooksey exercises to help her with her left peripheral lesion.

Obviously with that kind of fear, as indeed some nasty experiences of such mishaps, it compromises the daily activity of such patients.

The quality of life is certainly compromised in many of these patients, if not outright miserable. This subject has been investigated by Jahn and colleagues (2010) who agreed that gait disturbances are amongst the more common symptoms in the elderly. Reduced mobility markedly impairs quality of life, and the associated falls increase morbidity and mortality. They reviewed the literature based on a selective search on the terms 'gait,' 'gait disorder,' 'locomotion,' 'elderly,' 'geriatric' and 'ageing' (2000–2011/2009) and the findings of the authors' own studies on gait changes in old age and on the functional brain imaging of gait control. They discovered that gait disturbances in the elderly are often of multifactorial origin. The relevant pathogenic factors include sensory deficits (visual, vestibular, somatosensory), neurodegenerative processes (cortical, extrapyramidal motor, cerebellar), toxic factors (medications, alcohol) and anxiety (primary or concerning falls). A clinically oriented classification of gait disorders is proposed, which, on the basis of the characterisation of gait and the accompanying clinical findings, enables identification of the etiological factors and points the way to rational therapy. They believe that the evaluation of elderly patients whose chief complaint is a gait disturbance should be directed towards the identification of specific deficits. This is the prerequisite for rational therapy, even when the problem is of multifactorial origin. The preservation of mobility, they agree, is important in itself and also because the ability to walk is closely correlated with cognitive performance.

We think this is an invaluable study, duly highlighting various parameters and variables attributable to the problem of imbalance in the elderly. It is simply fascinating to read the various definitions given for disequilibrium and the factors that help in the maintenance of balance. It is our observation too that removing even a single sensory component such as visual even auditory element makes the older folks unsteady on their feet.

Situation could be worse if they have mini-infarcts in their cerebral cortex, seen on an MRI, leading to mild to moderate degree of amnesia, forgetfulness and even loss of direction. If such a patient has a motor or cerebellar lesion leading to ataxia, the situation could be worse, and challenging in terms of management. Neurological care would obviously be required in some of them.

In a fast-moving world, we tend to forget that one day we may have to go through similar situations where we may become handicapped, disabled or moribund enough to rely on charity and compassion of others. Family units regrettably are no more there, and one has to rely on hired help. Horrible stories of the nursing homes and hospices are displayed almost daily on the national media, where the likes of Dr. Shipman continue to play the role of death angels without mercy or human feelings of pain and agony, helplessness and misery that such elderly folks go through.

Not long ago, a man who called himself 'Dr. Death' wanted to travel to the UK to promote his so-called sympathetic ways of killing the aged, the disabled and the helpless. Even the controversial Liverpool care pathway for palliative care raises many an eyebrow and leaves a lot to explain.

Death can be a blessing for someone in absolutely helpless situations, but it should not remain in the hands of mankind to terminate life at will. Likewise assisted prolongation of life also remains a controversial issue. These ethical debates are necessary for clearing away the doubts and arrive at the right decisions.

In medicine, much emphasis is laid upon the principles and practices of ethics, but alas not to much benefit to the poorly and the elderly. All religions and most secular philosophers have taught the same fundamental rule of moral values. It is mandated in the divine books as 'Bid good, forbid evil'.

Kantian philosophy of Deontology is simple, logical and universal. Bentham and Mill's Utilitarianism is the other moral philosophy, which has its strong proponents. It has many questionable aspects in view of some ethicists. Every physician, however, must study these philosophies and normative ethical principles to draw benefits from the masters, in his day-to-day life.

One of the pillars of medical ethics is justice. But justice is not the same as equality or parity. Justice can be either distributive or retributive. Distributive justice demands that a person must be compensated according to his effort, contribution and input. And that is the very basic parameter that can determine if justice is being delivered or not. There are many a lacunae that one witnesses in day-to-day practice, particularly in the field of research or health care of the vulnerable. A combination of knowledge and skills is usually useful for mankind but can also prove to be lethal. The best illustration of which is the development of the nuclear bomb from an otherwise extremely beneficial technology. It is the fulcrum of conscience upon which must rest the heavy loads of knowledge and skills. Conscience determines whether an act is good or evil. However, since conscience is an imperceptible and a non-palpable entity, it is mirrored through justice, which is a tangible, noticeable and visible entity. If an act is just, it is ethical and good; if unjust, it has to be evil and unethical and must be condemned (Zaidi et al. 1995).

Regrettably the realities of life are different in modern days. Ever since the demise of the term 'patient' and its substitution by a word 'client or a customer' and the word 'doctor to health provider', all fundamental rules of humanity, empathy, trust, confidentiality and mutual affection between the patient and the physician seem to have undergone a total change.

In order to achieve the desired ethical outcomes, the 'rights and obligations' must match. The patients as well as the physicians have equal rights, and both parties also have certain obligations to fulfil. It is necessary that the medical schools teach normative principle of ethics and their applications to their students. But it is also equally necessary that the common citizens and the beneficiaries of health services understand and appreciate certain moral values and observe a code of ethics.

Modern medicine has many kaleidoscopic shades, but not all of them are bright and pleasing. Rival forces have made the profession become defensive in many ways. The ageless profession has changed.

It is sad to see medicine fall from grace. It is degraded from the high altar of a noble profession to a common trade!

12.1   Epilogue

Vertigo is indeed a malady for all ages; a conundrum in many ways. It affects children as well as the elderly with equal menace. Several studies described in this book duly highlight the incidence and prevalence of vertigo in different regions and different people, but not enough data is available to fully comprehend the impact of this clinically debilitating condition, on day-to-day life.

Numerous causes have been described and discussed in the world literature. Meniere's disease is somehow considered to be an icon of vertigo, which may not be true. We have found that our main problem was benign paroxysmal positional vertigo. It affects mainly the elderly but not always as we found out that it is fairly common in young adults also. It has also been reported to affect the children.

We believe that vestibular migraine is underrated as a major contributor to the plight of patients suffering with vertigo. It is far commoner than many reports have described and deserves to be given its due status amongst the notable causes of vertigo. Yes, Meniere's is an important clinical condition and demands a thorough assessment as indeed long-term management, but migraine-related vertigo is a salient as well as silent contributor to the menace.

Then, there are other important causes that we should remember such as vestibular neuronitis, labyrinthitis, ototoxicity, drug induced and iatrogenic causes. Amongst the central causes, an acoustic neuroma must be kept in mind, particularly if one is dealing with a vertiginous patient with unilateral tinnitus, sensorineural hearing loss or indeed an assay entry in hearing. Multiple sclerosis is another cause that one must remember as it has a long-term effect on the patient's life.

The non-vestibular causes related to the CVS or the CNS are best managed by the relevant specialities.

History and a thorough clinical examination are the backbone of managing a case of vertigo. Audiometry is an essential and very basic investigation, routinely carried out in an ENT clinic. Vestibular investigations should be arranged when clinically indicated. Calorimetry is an essential part of vestibulometry. It has stood the test of time, though a fresh crop of tests are challenging it, but time alone will tell. Videonystagmography has overtaken the ENG, and further avenues are currently being explored to be even more precise in locating the lesion. These are exciting times for anyone interested in the management of vertigo. One thing that remains underinvestigated is the subject of epidemiology. More regional, national and global data is needed to truly understand the burden of disease and disability caused by vertigo.

It affects children as well as adults. In children, it is often misdiagnosed and perhaps misunderstood. In adults, there is still a great deal of confusion about the frequency of common causes. Ménière's disease somehow has become an icon of vertigo. It certainly requires a review. There are many more conditions which are more common. For instance, BPPV is certainly commoner than Meniere's and vestibular migraine may also be more frequent than Meniere's, but it waits to be duly recognised as a major entity.

As the world grows older by the day, many fresh problems appear to take up the forefront, such as imbalance leading to falls and other co-morbidities. Therefore, not just a more thorough clinical evaluation but also the role of imaging becomes increasingly important.

In the field of management, the emphasis is definitely shifting from medicinal treatment to rehabilitative measures. Surgery for vertigo has become almost a rarity. The days of heroic endolymphatic surgery or radical skull base surgery have gone into background. Only a few selected centres perform such surgeries. These are the days of conservation and conservative approach rather than radical surgery. These are also the days of the keyhole surgery.

The future direction may rest with the development of dedicated balance clinics, which should be adequately funded to conduct research as indeed manage these patients more effectively.

The lessons that we have learnt from managing vertigo in a busy ENT clinic in the university-affiliated hospitals in England are manifold. But we still have much to learn. As clinicians, we must have the knowledge, the skills and due confidence to reach a firm diagnosis and treat it.

Finally, we believe that the medical world needs to pay more attention to the silent but potent menace of vertigo.

References

Charney DS, Deutch AY, Krystal JH, Southwick SM, Davis M (1993) Psychobiologic mechanisms of post traumatic disorder. Arch Gen Psychiatry 50:294–305

Cioffi D (1991) Beyond attention strategies: a cognitive –perpetual model of somatic interpretation. Psychol Bull 109:25–41

de Silva P (1999) Cultural aspects of post-traumatic disorder. In: William Y (ed) Post-traumatic disorders, concepts and theories. Willey, Chichester/New York, pp 116–138

Hassan HS, Laura G, William Y (1999) Chapter 7 published. In: William Y (ed) Psychobiology of post traumatic stress disorders concepts and therapy. Willey, Chichester/New York

Jahn K, Zwergal A, Schniepp R (2010) Gait disturbances in old age – classification, diagnosis, and treatment from a neurological perspective. Dtsch Arztebl Int 107(17):306–316, 0012–1207 (30 Apr 2010)

Kirby SE, Yardley L (2008) Understanding psychological distress in Meniere's disease. A systemic review. Psychol Health Med 13:257–273

Kirby S, Yardley L (2009) Psychological aspects of Meniere's disease and how to manage them. ENT News 18(1):56–57

LeDoux JE (1992) Emotion and amygdale. In: Aggelton JA (ed) The amygdale: neurobiological aspects of emotion, memory and mental dysfunction. Wiley-Liss, New York

Slaone P, Blazer D, George L (1989) Dizziness in a community elderly population. J Am Geriatr Soc 37(2):101–108

Yardley L (1994) Vertigo and dizziness. Routledge, London/New York, p 41

Yardley L, Dibb B, Osborne G (2003) Factors associated with quality of life in Meniere's disease. Clin Otolaryngol Allied Sci 28:436–441

Zaidi SH, Jafri M, Niaz U, Jawed S (1995) Medical ethics in contemporary era. Royal Book Co, Karachi

Index

S.H. Zaidi, A. Sinha, *Vertigo*,
DOI 10.1007/978-3-642-36485-3, © Springer-Verlag Berlin Heidelberg 2013

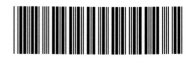